Geriatric Nutrition
and
Diet Therapy

by Marie Jaffe, R.N., M.S.

ISBN 0-944132-65-0

Published by Skidmore-Roth Publishing
1001 Wall Street
El Paso, Texas   79915

Printed in the United States of America

TABLE OF CONTENTS

CHAPTER I
GASTROINTESTINAL SYSTEM

ANATOMY AND PHYSIOLOGY

The gastrointestinal (GI) or digestive system consists of a hollow tubular structure that begins with the oral cavity and ends with the anus plus the associated organs that contribute to the digestion of nutrients. The primary function of the system is to supply nutrients to body cells, tissues and organs by ingestion (eating food), digestion (breaking down food), absorption (food transfer into circulation) and elimination (excretion of solid waste). It consists of the mouth, teeth and tongue, salivary glands (parotid, submaxillary and sublingual), pharnyx, esophagus, stomach, small intestine (duodenum, jejunum and ileum), pancreas, liver and gallbladder, large intestine (ascending, transverse and descending colon, rectum, anus). Nutrients, water, vitamins, minerals and electrolytes are received by the gastrointestinal tract and moved through it at a rate regulated by motility, secretions and absorption (see Fig. 1)

Innervation of the system is accomplished by the autonomic nervous system; the parasympathetic branch is excitatory and increases peristalsis and the sympathetic branch is inhibitory and decreases peristalsis.

The parts of the system and their functions are as follows:

1. **Oral cavity:** Receives food and begins preparation for absorption; teeth masticate the food to sizes appropriate for swallowing, tongue contains taste buds and positions food for swallowing, muscles for chewing that provide movement of food and larger surface area on which enzymes can act, salivary glands that secrete 1000-1500 ml/day contain salivary amylase (ptyalin) that begins the digestion of starches

2. **Pharnyx:** Closes the trachea as it assists in moving food into the esophagus

3. **Esophagus:** Connects the pharynx with the stomach and provides a passageway for the food facilitated by mucus secreting glands that lubricate the bolus of food as it passes along the tube by peristaltic waves. It is a 10 inch tube positioned behind the trachea that

contains a sphincter about 2 inches above entry into the stomach (cardiac sphincter). This entry remains closed unless peristaltic waves relax the sphincter allowing food to pass through to the stomach

4. **Stomach:** A hollow, pouchlike organ that stores the food early in the digestive process. Glands in the stomach secrete pepsinogen (chief cells) that digest protein, hydrochloric acid and the intrinsic factor glycoprotein (parietal cells) and mucus (mucous neck cells). About 2000 ml/day of gastric juices is secreted to mix with food and form chyme which is propelled into the duodenum of the small intestine in small amounts by peristalsis (every 15 - 25 seconds). The pyloric sphincter at the entrance to the duodenum prevents chyme from returning to the stomach. Blood supply to the stomach comes from the celiac artery and gastric veins which connect and terminate in the portal vein, draining venous blood. Gastrin is a hormone secreted by the antrum of the stomach and duodenum that stimulates the secretion of pepsinogen and hydrochloric acid, blood flow and smooth muscle contractions. Enzymes found in gastric juices include lipase, amylase, urease, lysozyme and carbonic anhydrase

5. **Small intestine:** The portion of the tract about 12 feet long that consists of the duodenum, jejunum and ileum and secretes about 3000 ml/day of digestive juices from the cells in the mucosa as well as the hormones cholecystokinin, enterogastrone, and secretin. It is here that chyme is further broken down, mixed and propelled from the stomach to the large intestine. Digestion and absorption mainly takes place in this part of the tract. The peristaltic activity that occurs here produce from 9-12 movements/minute and serve to mix the chyme with enzymes and bile which breaks down the substances to simpler forms for absorption by diffusion through the wall to the capillary beds. Blood supply to the small intestine comes from the gastroduodenal, celiac and pancreaticoduodenal arteries and the superior

3

mesenteric vein which empties into the portal vein and the liver drains the venous blood. The circulatory system carries the diffused nutrients to the body cells.

6. **Liver:** The largest gland in the body weighing about 3 pounds and secreting about 1000 ml bile/day. Its metabolic functions include protein, carbohydrate and fat metabolism, detoxification of drugs and steroid metabolism. It serves as a storage place for glucose, vitamins, fatty acids, amino acids and minerals among its other functions not related to the digestive system. The gallbladder concentrates and stores the bile secreted by the liver and releases it into the cystic duct and common bile duct into the duodenum for the process of digestion. It is reduced to urobilinogen by bacterial action and eliminated in the feces.

7. **Pancreas:** A gland whose exocrine acini cells secrete digestive juices and endocrine islet cells secrete hormones involved in glucose metabolism. The pancreatic digestive juices and enzymes aid in the digestion of proteins, carbohydrates and fats; the Islets of Langerhans secrete insulin by beta cells and glucagon by alpha cells and aid in the metabolism of glucose. Microscopic ducts empty into the pancreatic duct which empties into the duodenum carrying the pancreatic juices and enzymes needed for digestion. Insulin enters the portal circulation and travels to the liver where it is utilized or degraded. It assists in glucose storage, prevents breakdown of fat and increases synthesis of protein. An imbalance between insulin availability and insulin need that creates protein, carbohydrate and fat metabolism dysfunction is known as diabetes mellitus.

8. **Large intestine:** The portion of the tract about 5 feet long that consists of the cecum, ascending colon, transverse colon, descending colon, sigmoid colon, rectum and anal canal. Its major functions are the aborption of water and electrolytes and the formation of feces. It extends from the ileum to the anus and

retains feces by the sphincter ani. The glands secrete mucus that protects the bowel lining and provides lubrication for the mvoement of feces. Fecal mass is moved along the tract by peristalsis and eliminated when the rectal walls distend increasing intraabdominal pressure and relaxing the external sphincter. The consistency of the feces is determined by water absorption (usually 2000-3000 ml/day). Blood supply to the large intestine comes from the superior and inferior mesenteric arteries

THE GASTROINTESTINAL SYSTEM

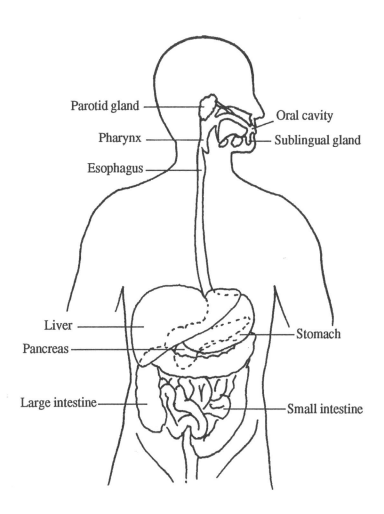

Fig. 1

LOCATION OF GASTROINTESTINAL ORGANS

RIGHT UPPER QUADRANT
Gallbladder
Duodenum
Head of pancreas
Lobe of liver
Upper part of kidney
Pylorus of stomach

LEFT UPPER QUADRANT
Lobe of liver
Spleen
Kidney
Stomach
Body of pancreas
Left transverse colon

RIGHT LOWER QUADRANT
Lower part of kidney
Cecum
Ascending colon
Appendix

LEFT LOWER QUADRANT
Sigmoid colon
Descending colon

CENTRAL ABDOMEN
Small intestines
(Duodenum, jejunum, ileum)

GASTROINTESTINAL HORMONES

HORMONES	SITE	STIMULUS	ACTION
Cholecystokinin	Duodenum	Fats	Stimulation of pancreas to produce enzymes and gallbladder to contract and release bile
Enterogastrone	Small Intestine	Fats, sugars, acids in the intestine	Inhibits gastric motility and secretion and relaxes sphincter of Oddi
Gastrin	Stomach, duodenum	Amino acids, alcohol, acid content in stomach, vagal stimulation	Stimulation of acid, pepsinogen secretion, blood flow and smooth muscle contraction (motility)
Secretin	Duodenum	Polypeptides and acidity of chyme	Stimulation of pancreas and liver to produce solution of bicarbonate (HCO_3-); inhibits motility

GASTROINTESTINAL ENZYMES

ENZYME	SITE	ACTION	END PRODUCT
Pytalin (salivary amylase)	Salivary glands	Starch	Polysaccharides
Pepsin	Stomach chief cells	Protein	Polypeptides
Gastric lipase	Stomach	Triglycerides	Glycerides

Enterokinase	Duodenum	Trypsinogen	Trypsin
Trypsin	Pancreas	Protein and poly-peptides	Polypeptides
Chymotrypsin	Pancreas	Other proteins and polypeptides	Polypeptides
Pancreatic lipase	Pancreas	Triglycerides	Glycerides, glycerol
Pancreatic amylase	Pancreas	Starch	Disaccharide, maltose
Aminopeptidase	Intestines	Polypeptides	Peptides
Dipeptidase	Intestines	Dipeptides	Amino acids
Maltase	Intestines	Maltose	Glucose
Lactase	Intestines	Lactose	Glucose, galactose
Intestinal lipase	Intestines	Fats	Glycerides, glycerol

ABSORPTION SITES

INTAKE	SITE
Protein	Jejunum
Carbohydrate	Jejunum
Fat	Jejunum
Vitamins	Duodenum (B_{12} in ileum)
Minerals	Small intestine
Water	Small and large intestine

9

GASTROINTESTINAL CHANGES RELATED TO THE AGING PROCESS

Alterations in the digestive process affected by the aging process include changes in secretion, reduction of nutrients, absorption, transport or motility. Nervous system changes also contribute to control organic functions by its sensory and motor losses which affect peripheral nerve conduction, its parasympathetic and sympathetic functions which affect intestinal motility and enzymatic release, its decreased vasomotor response which affects ingestion. A major number of complaints made by the elderly involve the gastrointestinal system beginning with the mouth and ending with the process of bowel elimination. The risk for digestive disorders are brought about from obstructive processes, absorption problems, vascular abnormalities and neurological changes in the aged population.

GENERAL GASTROINTESTINAL CHANGES ASSOCIATED WITH THE AGING PROCESS

Organ Structure/Anatomy

1. Teeth enamel thins causing teeth to become brittle

2. Grinding surface of teeth wears down causing decreased force of biting and chewing impairment

3. Bone loss in oral structures causing difficulty in fitting dentures, chewing food and decreasing tooth support

4. Thinning and drying of oral epithelium causing easily irritated and damaged mucous membranes

5. Increasing body fat and decreasing lean body mass. Changes in fat distribution with decreases in extremities and increases in abdomen and hips

6. Gradual weight decreases; with women decreases declining slower than men

7. Decreased subcutaneous tissue causing difficulty in environmental temperature adjustment

8. Decrease in liver size; pancreatic atrophy causing a decrease in exocrine cells for enzyme production

9. Alveolar degeneration and obstruction of the ducts of the pancreas causing blockage of secretions

10. Decreased mucosal surface area of small intestines causing altered absorption of nutrients

11. Atrophy of mucosa, muscle layers, arteriolar sclerosis, delay in peripheral nerve transmission of colon causing constipation or fecal incontinence

12. Weakness of abdominal and pelvic muscles causing difficulty in defecation

Physiologic Function

1. Reduced saliva production causing dry mouth and potential for breakdown of oral mucosa

2. Reduced number of taste buds causing altered taste and reduced food intake

3. Change in pH of saliva from acidic to alkalinic causing increased tendency for tooth decay

4. Decreased gag reflex causing swallowing difficulty

5. Decreased peristaltic activity and relaxation of smooth muscle of lower esophagus causing delayed emptying, dilitation and reflux

6. Decreased pepsin, hydrochloric acid secretion, intrinsic factor by stomach with a thinner mucosa and atrophic changes in the mucosa causing reduced absorption of vitamins B_1, B_2, B_{12}

7. Reduced pytalin with reduced saliva and reduced lipase and mucin secretion by stomach causing slowing of digestive process

8. Decreased metabolic rate causing weight gain

9. Decreased hepatic enzyme concentration causing a

reduced enzyme response to drug metabolism and detoxification

10. Bile thicker, contains higher cholesterol concentration and reduced in volume with emptying more difficult causing biliary tract disease (cholelithiasis) and obstruction with a decrease in fat soluble vitamin absorption by bile

11. Decreased secretion of amylase, lipase and trypsin by pancreas causing impaired digestion of lipids and splitting of large polypeptides into peptides which are acted upon in a singular fashion by the small intestine

12. Decreased absorption of nutrients by small intestine and reduced transport mechanism efficiency

13. Decreased enzyme secretion causing increased time required for digestion and reduced bacterial flora in large intestine

14. Decreased bowel motility, gastrocolic reflex, voluntary contraction of the external sphincter, amount of feces which all contribute to constipation or fecal incontinence

15. Vasculature of digestive tract (atherosclerosis) causing decreased blood supply of nutrients to bowel and possibly tissue injury

16. Decreased hunger contractions causing delayed gastric emptying

17. Decreased muscle tone and peristalsis of the bowel causing constipation and potential for obstruction

18. Increased swallowing of air when eating causing distention and eructation

PHYSIOLOGY FLOW SHEET

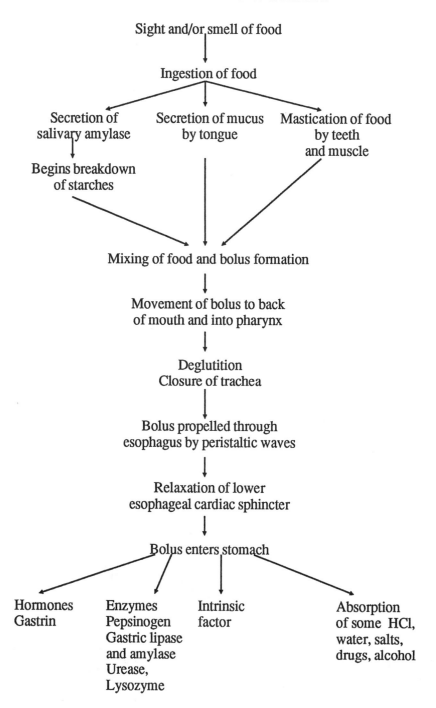

Sight and/or smell of food

Ingestion of food

Secretion of salivary amylase

Secretion of mucus by tongue

Mastication of food by teeth and muscle

Begins breakdown of starches

Mixing of food and bolus formation

Movement of bolus to back of mouth and into pharynx

Deglutition
Closure of trachea

Bolus propelled through esophagus by peristaltic waves

Relaxation of lower esophageal cardiac sphincter

Bolus enters stomach

Hormones
Gastrin

Enzymes
Pepsinogen
Gastric lipase
and amylase
Urease,
Lysozyme

Intrinsic
factor

Absorption
of some HCl,
water, salts,
drugs, alcohol

13

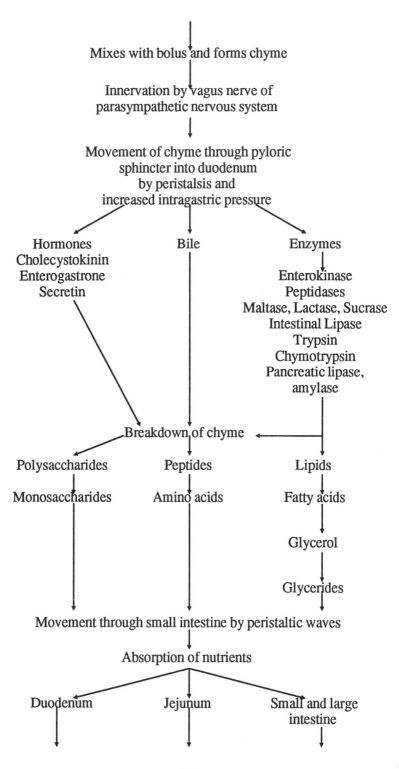

Mixes with bolus and forms chyme

Innervation by vagus nerve of
parasympathetic nervous system

Movement of chyme through pyloric
sphincter into duodenum
by peristalsis and
increased intragastric pressure

Hormones
Cholecystokinin
Enterogastrone
Secretin

Bile

Enzymes

Enterokinase
Peptidases
Maltase, Lactase, Sucrase
Intestinal Lipase
Trypsin
Chymotrypsin
Pancreatic lipase,
amylase

Breakdown of chyme

Polysaccharides

Monosaccharides

Peptides

Amino acids

Lipids

Fatty acids

Glycerol

Glycerides

Movement through small intestine by peristaltic waves

Absorption of nutrients

Duodenum

Jejunum

Small and large
intestine

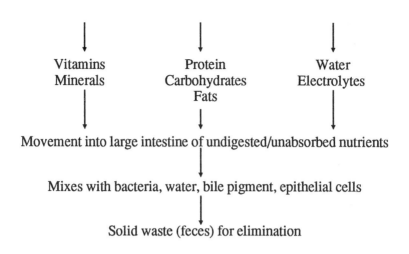

Vitamins Minerals	Protein Carbohydrates Fats	Water Electrolytes

Movement into large intestine of undigested/unabsorbed nutrients

Mixes with bacteria, water, bile pigment, epithelial cells

Solid waste (feces) for elimination

CHAPTER II
GASTROINTESTINAL/NUTRITIONAL ASSESSMENTS

AGE-RELATED TIPS FOR HISTORY INTERVIEW

1. The elderly have a high regard for privacy, use a private room or pull curtain when taking history

2. Greet client, shake hands if appropriate and address by title and name

3. Inform client of what is happening or about to happen and the length of the interview to promote trust and prevent apprehension and confusion

4. Speak and respond to client using words reflecting the age without infantilizing as this creates anxiety and anger in the elderly

5. Face client, maintain eye contact, speak in quiet, low and slow voice and accentuate consonants; use simple language and short words as elderly have decreased visual and auditory perception as a result of neurologic changes (be sure hearing aid is turned on if present and glasses are worn for increased acuity)

6. Ask one question at a time, repeat if necessary and allow time for response as elderly are slower to respond as result of decreased number of neurons

7. Avoid lengthy interviewing, perform comprehensive history taking over several interactions as the elderly have decreased energy reserves

8. Utilize touch during interview as this indicates warmth and caring and is usually well received by the elderly; refrain if client doesn't like it

9. Supplement data base by interviewing family member or close friend if mental acuity impaired; however avoid concluding that client is confused when this is not the case

10. Be sensitive and empathetic to client regardless of wellness, illness or frailty status and refrain from making ageism remarks

GASTROINTESTINAL SYSTEM HISTORY

I. Biographical Data:

Name_____

Age_____ Sex_____ Marital Status_____

Children/Grandchildren _____

Occupation _____

Education _____

II. Complaint(s):

Anorexia _____	Taste _____
Smell _____	Nausea _____
Reflux _____	Vomiting _____
Diarrhea_____	Constipation_____
Pyrosis_____	Dysphagia_____
Eructation _____	Dyspepsia_____
Dentures _____	Sore Mouth_____
Toothache _____	Poor Fitting Dentures _____
Flatulence _____	Fecal Incontinence _____
Distention _____	Rigid Facial Muscles _____
Hematemesis_____	Other_____

III. Past, Present Medical Status:

Gastrointestinal Surgeries _____

Diabetes_____	Hypertension _____
Thyroid Dysfunction_____	Ulcer_____
Hemorrhoids _____	Hiatal Hernia _____
Diverticulosis _____	Anemia_____
Heart Disease _____	Osteoporosis_____
Malnutrition _____	Cholecystitis_____

Dehydration_____ Accidents/Falls _____

Intestinal Infections/Inflammations_____

Chronic Renal Failure _____ Other _____

IV. Social Habits:

Alcohol _____ Smoking _____

Caffeine Beverages _____ Other _____

V. Psychological Factors:

Anxiety _____ Depression _____

Grieving_____ Boredom _____

Dementia _____ Disengagement _____

Communication Problem __ Loneliness_____

Other _____

VI. Special Considerations:

Special Diet _____

Food/Drug Allergies _____

Dental Hygiene Pattern _____

Use of Laxatives, Enemas and Type _____

Prescribed Medications _____

Exercise/Fatigue Pattern _____

Other _____

AGE-RELATED TIPS FOR PHYSICAL EXAMINATION

1. Provide privacy for all aspects of the physical assessment; use appropriate draping to ensure privacy and warmth as elderly chill easily

2. Relate normal physiologic aging changes of the system to findings

3. Allow client to empty bladder before examination to prevent accidental loss of urine

4. Place in prone position unless head elevation needed to facilitate breathing and chest expansion

5. Warm hands and stethoscope before touching client as elderly have reduced cold tolerance

6. The abdominal wall is thinner and more relaxed from loss of muscle tone and mass allowing for easier and more accurate palpation

7. The abdomen should be ausculatated prior to palpation or percussion to prevent changes in bowel sounds; use the diaphragm of the stethoscope for auscultation of bowel sounds

8. Examine all four quadrants of the abdomen and count sounds as this reveals bowel motility which is reduced in the elderly

9. The liver edge is more easily palpated in the elderly because of flattening of the diaphragm

10. The elderly may experience less pain and abdominal rigidity in acute or chronic conditions; abdominal distention is a common distress sign in the elderly

11. Physical assessment of the elderly gastrointestinal system should begin with the mouth and end with the anus

PHYSICAL ASSESSMENT

AREA	METHOD	NORMAL FINDINGS	ABNORMAL FINDINGS
Lips	Inspection	Pink, deeper vertical markings Symmetry during rest or movement	Red, pale or bluish Dry, cracked, chaffed Inflamed fissures at corners Lesions, ulcerations
Oral Mucosa	Inspection with tongue blade and penlight	Light or dark pink Thin, shiny mucosa	White or gray patches Redness, swelling, bleeding, exudate Sore mouth Irritated mucosa Lesions, ulcerations Dry mouth, halitosis
Gums	Same as above	Pink Gums/tooth margin tight	Red or pallor Bleeding on pressure Spurs, uneven ridges Lesions, ulcerations Pockets at tooth margins Swelling, pain
Tongue	Same as above	Pink, moist, shiny Symmetry, smooth and even with fissures	Red, swollen Lesion, patches Induration, limpness Lateral movement Sublingual varicosities

White exudate

Teeth	Same as above	Yellowish Firmly set Increased exposure of neck or teeth	Tooth loss Loose or broken teeth Wearing/erosion of teeth Toothache Periodontal disease Partial or full dentures
Pharynx	Same as above with gentle compression to back of tongue	Midline uvula Pink, smooth Tonsils present or absent	Uvula in lateral position Hypertrophied tonsils Swelling, exudate, redness of tonsils Lesions, plaques
Abdomen	Inspection	Pink but paler than other parts Smooth and soft Silvery striae Scars from surgeries Umbilicus in center Flat, rounded, concave contour Increased fat deposits Abdominal symmetry Smooth, even movements with breathing No visible peristalsis or pulsations	Jaundice, redness Bruises, cyanosis Lesions, rashes Skin taut, shiny Increased abdominal girth Umbilicus displacement Visible hernia Abdominal distention Concavity with wasting Bulges or masses in any area Increased, labored respirations with restricted abdominal movement Marked pulsations and visible peristalsis

Auscultation with stethoscope diaphragm in all four quadrants	Usually 5 to 34/ minute Sounds vary with gurgles, clicks, soft bubbling every 5-15 seconds	Absence of sound for 5 minutes Infrequent sounds Rapid, high-pitched tinkling noises Loud, gurgling noises
Auscultation with stethoscope bell	Absence of vascular sounds in epigastric, liver or spleen areas	Bruits (high-pitched, soft and swishing over artery) Venous hum (low-pitched, soft and continuous)
	Absence of friction rub over liver or spleen	Friction rub (like the sound of sandpaper rubbed together)
Percussion in all four quadrants	Dull to flat to tympanic depending on air or solid material in bowel Dullness over distended bladder	Dullness in any area or shifting dullness
	Upper and lower liver borders and liver span and movement within normal parameters	Enlarged liver with lower and upper borders span exceeding normal placement
	Small area of dullness or tympany over spleen	Enlarged spleen with extension of dullness or tympany changing to dullness on inspiration
Palpation, light and deep	Lax muscle tone No tenderness except deep palpation over cecum or sigmoid	Rigidity or resistance Deep visceral pain or cutaneous pain

		Normal	Abnormal
		Smooth feeling with consistent tension	Distention
		Slight inversion or eversion of umbilicus	Bulging or mass at umbilicus
		Palpable aorta, feces in colon, palpable femoral pulse	Mobile or fixed masses
		Liver border smooth and non-tender if felt on inspiration	Enlarged, nodular, irregular, tender liver
		Spleen non-palpable	Tenderness at splenic area
		Kidneys rarely palpable	Enlarged kidney
		Small, mobile, soft and smooth inguinal nodes	Tender, enlarged nodes
Rectum	Inspection	Course skin with no tenderness	Lumps, irritation, redness, hemorrhoids, soreness, scars, mucosa bulging through anus, tags, fissures
	Palpation	Smooth, even pressure on finger, smooth surface of rectal wall	Nodules, masses, loss of sphincter muscle tone Tenderness Fecal impaction
Feces	Inspection Guaiac test	Soft, brown	Black, tarry, chalky, Blood, pus, mucus Occult blood Loose, watery

PHYSICAL ASSESSMENT CHECKLIST

Name _____

Age_____ Ht_____ Wt_____ Frame _____

Abdominal girth_____ Skinfold thickness/Site_____

Inspection (note abnormalities):

Lips:_____ Gums:_____ Tongue: _____

Teeth:_____ Oral Mucosa: _____

Pharynx:_____ Abdomen:_____ Rectum: _____

Stool and characteristics: _____

Auscultation (note abnormalities):

Bowel sounds:_____Vascular sounds: _____

Percussion (note abnormalities):

Abdomen:_____ Bladder:_____ Liver:_____ Spleen: _____

Palpation (note abnormalities):

Abdomen:_____ Bladder:_____ Liver:_____ Spleen: _____

Rectum:_____ Anus: _____

Changes related to nutritional imbalances:

Eyes:_____ Hair:_____ Skin:_____ Nails: _____

Mucous membranes:_____ Skeletal:_____

Teeth:_____Muscles: _____

NOTES:

_____

_____

_____

_____

AGE-RELATED TIPS TO PROMOTE NUTRITION

1. Respect the food habits and preferences of the client; they reflect values, beliefs, culture and emotional status of an individual and have been developed over many years by the elderly

2. Behavior such as complaints, rejection or overeating is communicating an underlying problem

3. Be positive and show enthusiasm and encouragement at mealtime

4. Prepare client before meal time; provide mouth care, wash hands and face, place in sitting position; make sure teeth are in

5. Allow time for eating meal at slow pace; avoid facial expressions that convey hurriedness

6. Encourage self-feeding but assist in cutting meat, opening cartons and packages, protecting clothing when needed

7. Express attitude of a task that is important and worth your time when feeding a client

8. Allow for and accept feelings of frustration, anger and embarrassment

9. Provide adaptive aids for eating to those needing them

10. Provide food consistency and texture appropriate for chewing, swallowing problems

11. Maintain an environment free of odors, clean and orderly with appropriate temperature and ventilation

12. Encourage to chew foods well, eat slowly, take small bites at one time and explain how this aids digestion

13. Encourage intake of a moderate amount of fluids with meal and explain how this aids digestion and elimination

14. Avoid judgemental attitude regarding ethnic food habits or vegetarians

15. Be aware of the effect of drugs and emotional status on the nutritional well-being of the elderly (depression, loneliness, anxiety)

16. Common physical factors influencing nutrition are tooth pain and loss, reduced sense of smell and taste, reduced secretion of saliva and digestive juices and enzymes, decreased peristalsis, chronic diseases, physical handicaps

17. Communal meals reduce social isolation and loneliness; encourage to eat out of bed

18. Be aware of any dietary modifications related to a medical condition and offer food exchanges according to preferences, physical factors and appetite

19. Provide meals at intervals that will benefit client; 3 meals/day, 3 meals/day with between meal feedings, 6 meals/day, feedings every 2-4 hours

20. Request family to bring seasonings and special foods eaten at home

21. Avoid interruptions at mealtime for medications or procedures

22. Financial resources determine type and amount of food intake

23. Offer a variety of foods as monotony of foods cause loss of interest in eating

24. If living alone, bright colored meals and tablecloth, radio or TV during meals make mealtime more enjoyable

NUTRITIONAL ASSESSMENT

Name_____ Age___ Sex___ Date ____

Height_____ Weight_____ Frame _____

Recent Loss_____ Recent Gain _____

Minimum, Average and Maximum Weight in Past Month

_____

Chronic Disease(s) _____

Special Dietary Modifications _____

Special Ethnic/Cultural Considerations _____

Food/Drug Allergies_____ Prescribed Drugs_____

Food Preferences_____

_____

Food Rejections _____

_____

Eating Habits:

Attitude_____ Snacks_____ Eat Alone _____

Interest_____Meals/Day_____ Time of Meals _____

Amount of Food Consumed/Meal_____ 24 Hours_____

Calculated Caloric Need/24 Hours _____

Protein_____ Fat_____ Carbohydrate _____

Amount of Fluid Intake/24 Hours_____

Calculated Fluid Need/24 Hours_____

Nutritional Supplement_____ Vitamin/Mineral _____

Eating Problems:

Fatigue_____ Dentition/Dentures_____ Chewing _____

Swallowing____ Pyrosis____ Anorexia____ Dyspepsia____

Dry Mouth____ Ability to Feed Self____ Use of Aids _____

Disabilities:

Paralysis_____ Hand-Arm Coordination_____ Visual _____

29

Olfactory/Gustatory_____ Thirst Impairment_____

Alternative Feeding/Elimation Patterns:

Gastrostomy_____ Nasogastric Tube _____

Total Parenteral Nutrition _____

Intravenous Fluids_____ Colostomy_____

24 HOUR FOOD INTAKE

MEAL/TIME   FOOD   AMOUNT   CALORIES

Breakfast

Lunch

Dinner

Snacks

TOTAL

Total calculated recommended calories _____

Over/Under caloric requirement and amount _____

Number of Servings	Dairy Products	Meats	Vegetable/ Fruit	Bread/ Cereal	Candies Alcohol

BASIC 4/5 COMPARISON AND NEEDS _____

CHAPTER III
NUTRITIONAL PROBLEMS FOR NURSING CARE PLAN INCLUSION

NUTRITIONAL CARE PLANS FOR THE ELDERLY

- **Altered nutrition: less than body requirements**

Related factor: Inability to ingest food

Defining characteristics: Lack of interest in food

                            Reduced intake of calories and protein

                            Reduced olfactory/gustatory perception

                            Dysphasia

                            Anorexia

                            Nausea, vomiting

                            Sore mouth

                            Poor fitting dentures, toothache

                            Difficulty chewing

                            Abdominal distention

                            Early satiety

                            Loneliness/depression

                            Abdominal pain

                            Weight loss

Related factor: Inability to digest food

Defining characteristics: Reduced secretion of digestive enzymes and secretions

                            Vitamin/mineral deficiency

                            Surgeries such as gastric resection, small or or large bowel resection

                            Hepatitis, cirrhosis, pancreatitis

                            Common bile duct obstruction

                            Delayed gastric emptying

Related factor: Inability to absorb nutrients

Defining characteristics: Diarrhea

                            Inadequate absorbing surface (surgery of small, large bowel)

                            Abnormal bowel motility

                            Bacterial overgrowth (anti-infectives)

                            Malnutrition

                            Vascular insufficiency and reduced circulation to gastrointestinal organs

- Altered nutrition: more than body requirements

Related factor:	Excessive intake in relationship to metabolic need
Defining characteristics:	Weight at least 10% over ideal for height, frame
	Decreased metabolic rate
	Sedentary activity level
	Increased intake
	Dysfunctional eating pattern (response to internal and external cues other than hunger)

- Altered oral mucous membrane

Related factor:	Dehydration
	Ineffective oral hygiene
	Periodontal disease
	Poor fitting dentures
	Decreased salivation, xerostomia
	Thinning and drying of oral epithelium
	Mouth breathing
	Decreased sensation to hot/cold foods
	Malnutrition
	Nasogastric tube
Defining characteristics:	Oral burns, lesions
	Xerostomia
	Oral pain or discomfort
	Halitosis
	Redness, irritation of mucosa, gums
	Bleeding from gums
	Coated tongue

- Altered tissue perfusion (gastrointestinal)

Related factor:	Interruption of arterial flow
Defining characteristics:	Decreased circulation to digestive organs
	Nausea, vomiting
	Poor nutrition

- Bowel incontinence

Related factor:	Neuromuscular involvement
	Musculoskeletal involvement
	Anxiety, depression
	Impaired sensory perception (tactile)

Defining characteristics:	Involuntary passage of stool
	Lack of awareness of urge to defecate
	Stained clothing
	Use of protective pads, underwear

- Constipation

Related factor:	Less than adequate intake, bulk/fiber intake
	Less than adequate fluid intake
	Less than adequate physical activity or immobility
	Medications/habitual use of laxatives
	Neuromuscular impairment
	Musculoskeletal impairment
	Emotional status
Defining characteristics:	Frequency less than usual pattern
	Hard-formed stool
	Excessive straining during elimination
	Decreased bowel sounds
	Less than usual amount of stool
	Abdominal discomfort, distention
	Flatulence
	Fecal impaction

- Diarrhea

Related factor:	Stress and anxiety
	Dietary intake
	Medications (anti-infectives, laxatives)
	Malabsorption of bowel
	Bowel inflammation
Defining characteristics:	Abdominal cramping
	Increased frequency
	Loose, liquid stools
	Urgency
	Changes in color and odor of stool
	Increased motility/bowel sounds
	Positive stool culture for toxins, causative microorganism
	Temperature elevation

- High risk for aspiration

Related risk:	Decreased gag reflex
	Decreased peristalsis activity and relaxation of lower esophagus sphincter
	Reduced level of consciousness
	Gastrointestinal feeding tube
	Increased gastric residual
	Delayed gastric emptying
	Impaired swallowing
	Decreased gastrointestinal motility
Defining characteristics:	Choking, coughing
	Vomiting, nausea
	Dysphagia
	Aspiration pneumonia

- High risk for fluid deficit

Related risk:	Extremes of age
	Excessive losses through diarrhea, vomiting, other normal routes
	Loss of fluid through indwelling tubes, other abnormal routes
	Inability to secure fluids (immobility)
	Medication (diuretics)
	Altered intake
	Impaired thirst sensation
Defining characteristics:	Increased fluid output
	Decreased fluid intake
	Dehydration
	Electrolyte imbalance
	Thirst, dry skin and mucous membranes
	Weight loss
	Decreased skin turgor
	Weakness
	Temperature elevation

- Impaired swallowing

Related factor:	Neuromuscular impairment
	Fatigue
	Limited awareness
Defining characteristics:	Absent gag reflex
	Inability to chew food

Rigidity of facial muscles
Coughing/choking
Stasis of food in oral cavity

- Knowledge deficit
Related factor: Lack of recall, exposure to information
                              Cognitive limitation
                              Lack of interest in learning
                              Requests no information
Defining characteristics: Communication impairment
                              Intellectual impairment
                              Agitation, apathy
                              Inability to perform ADL or manage own
                              medical regimen

- Self-care deficit, feeding
Related factor: Neuromuscular impairment
                              Depression
                              Disorientation
                              Cognitive impairment
Defining characteristics: Inability to feed self or manipulate utensils
                              Paralysis
                              Unable to use assistive aid
                              Unable to lift glass to mouth
                              Unable to cut meat, butter bread
                              Reduced state of consciousness

- Sensory/perceptual alterations
Related factor: Aging
                              Chronic illness
                              Altered status of sense organs
                              (olfactory/gustatory)
                              Sleep deprivation
                              Medications
Defining characteristics: Change in taste and smell
                              Disorientation
                              Apathy, anxiety
                              Change in behavior pattern

CHAPTER IV

ESSENTIAL NUTRIENTS AND FUNCTIONS

BASIC FOOD GROUPS

FOOD GROUP	SERVINGS REQUIRED PER DAY	NUTRIENTS SUPPLIED
Dairy products	2 cups	Protein Vitamins A, D, B_6, B_{12} Calcium, phosphorus, zinc magnesium
Fruits and vegetables	4 servings that includes 1 of citrus fruit and 1 green or yellow vegetable	Carbohydrate Thiamin, niacin Vitamins A, C, B_6, E Phosphorus, magnesium, calcium, iron Fiber
Meat, fish, eggs, legumes, nuts	2 servings	Protein Thiamin, niacin, riboflavin Vitamins, A, E Iron, iodine, phosphorus, magnesium, zinc
Bread, cereals, grains, pasta, rice	4 servings	Complex carbohydrate Thiamin, niacin Vitamin B_6, E Magnesium, iron, zinc, folacin
Supplementary foods, condiments	No specific requirements, but should be considered in meal calculations and planning	Alcohol, chocolate, caffeine beverages, jams/jelly, candy, syrup, pastries, cookies, potato chips, snack foods, mayonnaise, butter, olives, margarine, seasonings, catsup, pickles, mustard, spices

RECOMMENDED DAILY DIETARY ALLOWANCES

SUBSTANCE	MALE (AGE 50+) WT 154 lb, HT 70 in	FEMALE (50+) WT 120 lb, HT 64 in
FOOD NUTRIENTS		
PROTEIN	56 gm or 0.8 gm/kg	44 gm
CARBOHYDRATE	50-55% of total calories/day	
FAT	30% of total calories/day	
CALORIES	2000-2400 total calories/day after age 55	

VITAMINS AND MINERALS

VIT. A	1000 mcg	800 mcg
VIT. B_1 (Thiamin)	1.2 mg	1.0 mg
VIT. B_2 (Riboflavin)	1.4 mg	1.3 mg
VIT. B_6 (Pyridoxine)	2.2 mg	2.2 mg
VIT. B_3 (Niacin)	16 mg	13 mg
VIT. B_{12} (Cyanocobalamin)	3.0 mcg	3.0 mcg
VIT. C (Ascorbic Acid)	60 mg	60 mg
VIT. D (Calciferol)	5 mcg	5 mcg
VIT. E (Tocopherol)	10 mg	8 mg
VIT. K	70-140 mcg	70-140 mcg
FOLACIN	400 mcg	400 mcg
BIOTIN	100-200 mcg	100-200 mcg
PANTOTHENIC ACID	4-4 mg	4-7 mg
CALCIUM	800 mg	800 mg
CHLORIDE	1700-5100 mg	1700-5100 mg
POTASSIUM	1875-5625 mg	1875-5625 mg
SODIUM	1100-3300 mg	1100-3300 mg
PHOSPHORUS	800 mg	800 mg
MAGNESIUM	350 mg	300 mg

MANGANESE	2.5-5.0 mg	2.5-5.0 mg
SELENIUM	0.05-0.2 mg	0.05-0.2 mg
COPPER	2.0-3.0 mg	2.0-3.0 mg
FLOURIDE	1.5-4.0 mg	1.5-4.0 mg
CHROMIUM	0.05-0.2 mg	0.05-0.2 mg
MOLYBDENUM	0.15-0.5 mg	0.15-0.5 mg
IRON	10 mg	10 mg
ZINC	15 mg	5 mg
IODINE	150 mcg	150 mcg

FOOD NUTRIENTS

The three main categories of foods are identified as proteins, carbohydrates and fats. Proteins, the building blocks, are composed of amino acids which may be essential or nonessential (essential cannot be synthesized and must come from food and nonessential are those that can by synthesized by the body to meet requirements). Carbohydrates, the provider of the most efficient forms of energy, are classified into monosaccharides, disaccharides and polysaccharides, and fats, the body's most concentrated source of energy, consist of fatty acids, triglycerides, cholesterol and phospholipids.

PROTEIN

RDA	0.8 Gm/kg/day (age and body size dependent)
Principle sources	Milk and milk products except butter, meat, fish, poultry, eggs, seafood, legumes
Functions in body	Tissue maintenance Formation of hormones, enzymes, antibodies Regulates fluid balance of cells and maintenance of blood neutrality (acid-base balance)
Deficiency	Wasting of muscle tissue, weight loss, delayed healing of wounds and fractures, edema, infection
Persons at risk	Elderly, malnutrition, immobility, vegetarianism
Comments	1 Gm protein = 4 kcal

CARBOHYDRATE

RDA
50-55% of total calories/day

Principle sources
Cereal grains, whole grains, fruit, vegetables, nuts, sugar and sweets, milk and milk products, dietary fiber

Functions in body
First substances to be used to produce energy
Regulator of body processes by its content in hormones, enzymes, nervous tissue, connective tissue, RNA, DNA
Indigestible portions promote bowel function

Deficiency
Metabolism of protein and fat for energy; breakdown of body tissues

Persons at risk
Diabetics, lactose intolerance

Comments
1 Gm = 4 kcal
Alcohol yields: 1 Gm = 7 kcal
Overconsumption of sugars lead to obesity, dental disease
Excess carbohydrate is stored as glycogen and body fat

FAT

RDA
30% of total calories/day

Principles sources
Milk and milk products, meat, fish, poultry, olives, avocados, nuts, seeds, oils, margarine

Functions in body
Concentrated source of energy in form of fatty acids
Insulates, cushions and protects body
Carries fat soluble vitamins

Deficiency
Dermatitis, disturbances in fat metabolism

Excess	Obesity, atherosclerosis
Persons at risk	Arterial insufficiency, hypertension, coronary artery disease, gallbladder, liver disease
Comments	1 Gm = 9 kcal Common terminology regarding fats include saturated, polyunsaturated and cholesterol

VITAMINS

A vitamin is an organic compound derived from the diet. Very small quantities are needed to promote growth and maintain life. The following provides information about the major vitamins (fat and water soluble) needed for a complete understanding of their functions, sources, adverse effects of deficiencies and toxicities and daily requirements for the older adult.

VITAMIN A (Fat Soluble)

RDA	5,000 IU or 1,000 mcg/day for male and 4,000 IU or 800 mcg/day for female
Principle sources	Egg yolk, liver, lamb, milk, butter, cheese , margarine Yellow-orange pigment foods: apricots, cantaloupe, peaches, carrots, sweet potatoes, yellow squash Green vegetables: broccoli, spinach
Function in body	Vision at night, mucous membranes and secretions, steroid hormone synthesis, formation of bone and cartilage growth and repair of cells, dental development, spermatogenesis
Storage in body	Liver
Overdose symptoms	Greater than 50,000 IU/day for 2-3 weeks; lethargy, anorexia, drying and desquamation of skin, headache, sweating, bone pain, jaundice, alopecia, photophobia, hepatomegaly, splenomegaly
Deficiency symptoms	Night blindness, spots, xerophthalmia, keratinization of epithelial tissue, hyperkeratosis
Persons at risk	Elderly; persons with diabetes, hyperthyroidism; alcoholics, smokers
Antagonists	Air pollution, strong light, mineral oil,

	increased protein intake
Synergists	Vitamins C, D and E
Comments	Carotine is the precursor to vitamin A, is fat soluble and insoluble in water and absorbed in the small intestine

VITAMIN D-CALCIFEROL (Fat Soluble)

RDA	200 IU or 5 mcg/day for male and female
Principle sources	Sunlight, liver oils, margarine, lard, egg yolks, butter, vitamin D milk, shrimp, salmon, tuna
Function in body	Growth and repair of bone; maintains calcium and phosphorus balance and absorption from intestine
Storage in body	Liver and skin
Overdose symptoms	1000-3000 IU/kg/day, calcification of skin, blood vessels and kidneys and other soft tissue, anorexia, diarrhea, polyuria, muscle weakness, kidney stones
Deficiency symptoms	Osteomalacia, hypothyroidism, tetany osteoporosis, tooth decay, decreased muscle tone
Persons at risk	Elderly; persons with lead poisoning or deprived of sunlight
Antagonists	Cortisone, anticonvulsants
Synergists	Vitamins A, B_1, B_3, C and calcium
Comments	Mild bone deformities; permanent serious derformities

VITAMIN E-TOCOPHEROL (Fat Soluble)

RDA

10 mg/day for male and 8 mg/day
for female

Principle sources

Vegetable oil, margarine, peanuts,
whole grains, chocolate, yeast, cabbage,
broccoli, asparagus, spinach

Function in body

Metabolism of fats
Antioxidant
Maintains cell membrane integrity
Prevention of premature aging
Protection against lung damage by
pollutants and smoking
Aids in stress response of body

Storage in body

Highest concentration in liver, pituitary
gland, testes and adrenal glands

Overdose symptoms

Possible increase in blood pressure,
interference with clotting function

Deficiency symptoms

Anemia, degeneration of reproductive
tissue and muscle, liver necrosis

Antagonists

Rancid fats and oils, iron if taken at same
time, mineral oil, thryoid hormone

Synergists

Vitamins A, B complex, C, cortisone,
testosterone, STH

Comments

Avoid taking with iron preparation

VITAMIN K(Fat Soluble)

RDA

70-140 mcg for male and female
reported but manufactured in the
intestine daily

Principle sources

Liver, kidney, beef, pork, spinach,
cauliflower, kale, green leafy vegetables

Functions in body	Synthesis of prothrombin and other blood clotting factors by the liver
Storage in body	Liver; produced daily by intestinal flora
Overdose symptoms	Vomiting, possible thrombosis, porphyrinuria
Deficiency symptoms	Hypoprothrombinemia, hemorrhage or tendency to bleed easily
Persons at risk	Those with chronic diarrhea or disorders that interfere with intestinal absorption
Antagonists	Anticoagulants, penicillin, tetracycline, sulfonamides, aspirin, mineral oil
Synergists	Vitamins A, C, E
Comments	Requires the presence of bile for its absorption that takes place in upper part of small intestine

VITAMIN B$_1$- THIAMIN (Water Soluble)

RDA	1.2 mg/day for male and 1.0 mg/day for female
Principle sources	Yeast, wheat germ, whole grains, pork, liver, plums, prunes, raisins, asparagus, corn, peas, rice, peanuts, beans, potatoes
Functions in body	Metabolism of carbohydrate, synthesis of acetylcholine for health of nerve fibers and neurons, and digestion
Storage in body	Very little stored; muscles, brain, kidneys, liver and heart have small amount of concentration
Overdose symptoms	Greater than 6000 mg/day; edema, tremors, tachycardia, fatty liver, sweating,

	hypotension
Deficiency symptoms	Nerve degeneration, fatigue, anorexia, weight loss, muscular atrophy, mental disturbances (depression)
Persons at risk	Alcoholics, post-surgical status, cardiac conditions, elderly, long term hemodialysis, chronic febrile conditions
Antagonists	Raw fish, tea, emotional stress, alcohol, antibiotics, nitrates, baking soda
Synergists	Vitamins B_2, B_3, B_6, B_{12}, C, D and pantothenic acid
Comments	Absorbed in the duodenun and jejunun Great amount loss in preparation of foods in water

VITAMIN B_2-RIBOFLAVIN (Water Soluble)

RDA	1.4 mg/day for male and 1.3 mg/day for female
Principle sources	Milk, meat, fish, poultry, whole grains, liver, heart, kidney, eggs, avocados, beans, asparagus, broccoli, corn, peas, spinach
Function in body	Maintenance of epithelium, eye, mucous membranes, part of respiratory enzymes, component of oxidases that oxidize fatty acids and amino acids
Storage in body	Stored mainly in liver and kidneys but increases above daily needs are excreted by the kidneys
Overdose symptoms	Essentially nontoxic
Deficiency symptoms	Angular stomatitis, glossitis, photophobia, conjunctivitis, seborrheic

dermatitis, cracks at mouth corners

Persons at risk	Chronic alcoholics, elderly, severe gastrointestinal diseases interferring with absorption, achlorhydria, hyperthyroidism
Antagonists	Antibiotics
Synergists	Vitamins A, B3, E
Comments	Absorbed rapidly in upper part of the small intestine
	Easily destroyed by alkali as in pasteurized milk, use of baking soda to preserve the green color in vegetables or in preparation of meat by baking

VITAMIN B3-NIACIN, NICOTINIC ACID, NICOTINAMIDE, NIACINAMIDE (Water Soluble)

RDA	16 mg/day for male and 13 mg/day for female
Principle sources	Liver, chicken, poultry, fish, yeast, peanuts, enriched grain products, most vegetables
Functions in body	Metabolism of proteins, carbohydrates and fats, pigment metabolism
	Synthesis of fatty acids and cholesterol
	Electron transport in cellular respiratory reactions
Storage in body	Heart, liver and muscles (limited) with any excess excreted by the kidneys
Overdose symptoms	3000 mg/day or more; flushing, burning and itching of skin, fatty liver, arrhythmias, gastrointestinal problems
Deficiency symptoms	Pellagra with dermatitis, diarrhea and

dementia, anorexia, weakness

Persons at risk	Alcoholics, hyperthyroidism, gastrointestinal conditions, diabetics
Antagonists	Antibiotics, emotional and physical stress
Synergists	Vitamins A, B_1, B_2, B_6, B_{12}, C, D
Comments	Absorbed in the smalll intestine Tryptophan is a precurson of B_3 and dependent on B_6 for the conversion

VITAMIN B_6-PYRIDOXINE, PYRIDOXAL, PYRIDOXAMINE (Water Soluble)

RDA	2.2 mg/day for male and female
Principle sources	Fish, poultry, meats, wheat germ, brown rice, peanuts, molasses, walnuts, soybeans, lima beans, yeast
Functions in body	Metabolism of proteins, carbohydrates and fats, synthesis of antibodies, erythrocyte formation
Storage in body	Some in leukocytes, nerve tissue and liver with excess excreted by kidneys as pyridoxic acid
Overdose symptoms	More than 1000 mg/day; limited toxicity responses
Deficiency symptoms	Seborrheic dermatitis, glossitis, angular stomatitis, peripheral neuropathy, anemia
Persons at risk	Chronic alcoholism, malabsorption syndromes
Antagonists	Isonicotine hydrazine, antihypertensives, levodopa, cortisone, penicillamine
Synergists	Vitamins B_1, B_2, B_3, C, magnesium

| Comments | Absorption not known but it is found in the extracellular fluid |
| | Included in RDA in 1968 |

VITAMIN B$_{12}$-COBALAMIN, CYANOCOBALAMIN (Water Soluble)

RDA	3.0 mcg/day for male and female
Principle sources	Lamb and beef kidney, lamb, beef, calf and pork liver, beef brain, egg yolk, clams, oysters, sardines, herring, salmon
Functions in body	Required by all cells especially bone marrow, nervous system and gastro-intestinal tract
	Synthesis of folacin and production of leukocytes
	Regulates formation of erythrocytes
Storage in body	In liver for 3-5 years
Overdose symptoms	No known toxic effects
Deficiency symptoms	Pernicious anemia (pallor, weight loss, glossitis, sprue, anorexia)
	Moodiness, memory loss
Persons at risk	Vegetarians, surgical removal of stomach, lack of intrinsic factor that prevents absorption of B$_{12}$
Antagonists	Aspirin, codeine, neomycin
Synergists	Vitamin A, B$_1$, C, E, folic acid, biotin, pantothenic acid
Comments	Cobalamin containing enzymes involved in the transfer of carbon units
	Defect in absorption caused by lack of intrinsic factor production by stomach

VITAMIN C-ASCORBIC ACID (Water Soluble)

RDA	60 mg/day for male and female
Principle sources	Fresh, frozen or raw fruits and vegetables
Functions in body	Conversion of folic acid to an active form Wound healing, aids in fighting infection, injury and stress Maintains body structure and metabolizes some amino acids Synthesis of steroids from cholesterol Reduction of ferric iron to ferrous iron for absorption Maintains capillaries, acts as an antioxidant
Storage in body	Found in adrenal glands, kidneys, spleen, liver, pancreas and pituitary and after tissues are saturated, the excess is excreted
Overdose symptoms	Edema, tremors, impaired WBC acivity, tachycardia, fatty liver, possible kidney stones and damage to pancreas, excessive iron absorption
Deficiency symptoms	Scurvy, aching joints and muscles, poor wound healing, muscular weakness, anorexia, ecchymoses, bleeding gums, loose teeth, petechiae
Persons at risk	Wounds or surgical incisions High levels of stress
Antagonists	Smoking, pollution, alcohol, aspirin, diuretics, prednisone, antidepressants, anticoagulants, indomethacin
Synergists	B complex vitamins, vitamins A, K, E, testosterone
Comments	Absorbed from the gastrointestinal tract

Easily destroyed by oxidation (prolonged cooking, exposure to iron, oxygen, copper, light, and alkali)
Slicing food releases oxidative enzymes from surfaces

FOLACIN-B Complex (FOLIC ACID, FOLATE)

RDA	400 mcg/day for male and female
Principle sources	Liver, asparagus, spinach, yeast, bran, dry beans, wheat, green leafy vegetables, corn, peanuts, oats, barley, walnuts
Functions in body	Synthesis of choline, DNA, RNA and amino acids. Coenzyme in purine, pyrimidine metabolism
Storage in body	Most stored in liver and excreted in urine and feces.
Overdose symptoms	No toxicity ever reported
Deficiency symptoms	Pernicious anemia, macrocytic anemia, sprue, glossitis, leukopenia, thrombocytopenia
Persons at risk	Alcoholics, leukemia, intestinal disorders elderly, Hodgkin's disease
Antagonists	Antimalarials, anticonvulsants, alcohol, sulfonamides, methotrexate
Synergists	B complex vitamins, vitamin C, testosterone, estradiol
Comments	Deficiency is usually concurrent with vitamin C deficiency Synthesized by intestinal flora

BIOTIN-B Complex

RDA	100-200 mcg/day for male and female
Principle sources	Liver, yeast, meats, seafood, nuts, corn, soybeans, eggs, mushrooms, chocolate
Functions in body	Metabolism of carbohydrates and fats and protein Maintenance of skin, hair, nerves and bone marrow
Storage in body	Small amounts in liver, kidneys, brain and adrenals with excretion in urine and feces
Overdose symptons	Nontoxic in humans
Deficiency symptoms	Muscle pain, anorexia, nausea, vomiting, glossitis, scaly skin, depression
Persons at risk	No reports
Antagonists	Raw egg white, antibiotics, sulfonamides
Synergists	B complex vitamins, vitamin A, D,
Comments	Synthesized by intestinal flora Stable to acids, heat and light Affected by alkaline solutions and oxidizing agents

PANTOTHENIC ACID-B Complex

RDA	4-7 mg/day for male and female
Principle sources	Liver, kidney, eggs, yeast, wheat germ, dried peas, peanuts, meats, cheese, clams, herring, salmon, mackerel, oats, soybeans, rice; widely distributed in foods
Functions in body	Cellular metabolism of proteins, fats,

and carbohydrates
Synthesis of fatty acids, steroids,
cholesterol, acetylcholine, porphyrin

Storage in body	Found in heart, liver, brain, kidneys and adrenal glands
Overdose symptoms	Nontoxic in humans
Deficiency symptoms	Not usual but can be induced; fatigue, malaise, numbness, muscle cramps, burning of feet, insomnia, nausea, abdominal cramping, indigestion, susceptibility to infection, impaired muscular coordination
Persons at risk	Wounds, physical or emotional stress
Antagonists	Insecticides
Synergists	B complex vitamins, vitamins A, C, E, calcium
Comments	Stable under ordinary cooking procedures except in acid or alkaline solutions Known as the anti-stress vitamin

MINERALS

Minerals are substances in the human body that are involved in hormonal activity, oxygen transport, maintenance of fluid and electrolyte balance, osmotic pressure, muscle contraction, the response of nerves to stimuli and many other functions that are necessary for life. Minerals are present in large amounts and trace amounts (trace elements).

CALCIUM (Ca)

RDA	800 mg/day for male and female
Principle sources	Milk and dairy products, spinach, mustard collard and turnip greens, shrimp, clams, oysters, salmon
Functions in body	Catalyst for conversion of prothrombin into thrombin, transmission of nerve impulses, activation of enzymes, control of integrity of cement substances and cell membranes
Storage in body	Body contains 1200-1250 Gm of Ca with 99% in bones and teeth

Most of the Ca eliminated is excreted in the feces with a small amount in urine; some is lost in sweat |
Overdose symptoms	Hypercalcemia, cardiac arrhythmias; lethargy, weakness, muscle flaccidity, headache, anorexia, nausea, vomiting; milk-alkali syndrome
Deficiency symptoms	Tetany (muscular twitching, tremors, paresthesia, spasmodic contractions), osteoporosis with spontaneous fractures
Persons at risk	Elderly, antacid and milk therapy for peptic ulcer, parathormone and calcitonin secretion dysfunction, vitamin D deficiency

Antagonists	High phosphorus diet
Synergists	Vitamin D, high protein diet, lactose
Comments	Absrobed in the duodenum as Ca salts more soluble in an acid medium
	30% of Ca in diet is absorbed by the adult
	Increased motility and achlorhydria decrease absorption

PHOSPHORUS (PO4)

RDA	800 mg/day for male and female
Principle sources	Milk and milk products, lean meats; found in most foods
Functions in body	Transports fat in blood
	Transport of substances in and out of cells
	Glucose absorption in the intestine and uptake by cells and resorption by renal tubules
	Storage and release of energy (ATP, ADP)
	Activates B vitamins
Storage in body	80-90% in bones and teeth with the remaining in all cells in form of phosphate ion (PO_4), eliminated in feces and urine
Overdose symptoms	Renal disease, hypoparathyroidism, hypocalcemia with tetany (muscular twitching, tremors, paresthesia), hyper-phosphatemia, poor urinary output
Deficiency symptoms	Malabsorption (sprue or celiac disease), bone disease (osteomalacia), muscle weakness, hypophosphatemia, malnutri-tion, hypercalcemia

Persons at risk	Kidney disease, parathyroid dysfunction
Antagonists	Iron, calcium, aluminum
Synergists	B vitamins, vitamin D, glucose
Comments	Absorption in the intestines after broken down by enzymes (phosphatases) Dietary phosphorus should equal calcium intake

MAGNESIUM (Mg)

RDA	350 mg/day for male and 300 mg/day for female
Principle sources	Whole grains, legumes, green leafy vegetables, seafood, nuts, cocoa
Functions in body	Catalyst for biological reactions Transmission of nerve impulses Active transport across cell membranes Muscle contractions Transfers ATP to a phosphate acceptor
Storage in body	About 20-35 Gm in body with 70% combined with calcium and phosphorus in bone; the remaining amount found in body fluids and within the cells and in muscle Eliminated in urine and feces
Overdose symptoms	More than 15 Gm/day; flushed feeling, muscular weakness, hypotension, diminished reflexes, perspiration, decreased urinary output; hyper-magnesemia
Deficiency symptoms	Hypomagnesemia, twitching, tremors, spasticity, restlessness, confusion, positive Chvostek's sign

Persons at risk	Chronic alcoholism, cirrhosis of liver, malabsorption, malnutrition, dehydration, diuretics, renal failure, antacids and laxatives containing magnesium
Antagonists	Excess fat, phosphates, oxalic and phylic acids
Synergists	Acidic environment, potassium
Comments	Absorption in the small intestine High intake of calcium increases requirement of magnesium

IRON (Fe)

RDA	10 mg/day for male and female
Principle sources	Fish and shellfish, beef, lamb, pork, veal, liver, kidney, ham, poultry, legumes, spinach, broccoli, green beans, cabbage, dried fruits, nuts, oats, barley, wheat germ, noodles
Function in body	Uptake and release of oxygen at cellular level and energy production
Storage in body	4 Gm iron in the body with majority found in the hemoglobin of erythrocytes; 1 Gm is stored in liver and spleen with the remaining stored in cells for ready use Losses occur in sweat, hair, sloughing of epithelial and mucosa and urine; bleeding and trauma add to iron loss
Overdose symptoms	More than 100 mg/day; poor liver function, diabetes from pancreas dysfunction, bronze skin, arrhythmias
Deficiency symptoms	Anemia, weakness, fatigue, pallor, dyspnea, tachycardia
Persons at risk	Malabsorption disorders, chronic blood

	loss, chronic renal failure, cancer of gastrointestinal tract, high altitudes
Antagonists	Tea, phosphates, oxalates and phytates, increased fiber intake
Synergists	Absorbic acid, fructose, sulfhydryl compounds, copper, acidic environment
Comments	Absorption in the small intestine Present in foods in form of heme or nonheme iron with heme iron found in animal tissues and nonheme in vegetable sources

IODINE (I)

RDA	150 mcg/day for male and female
Principle sources	Seafood, eggs, iodized salt
Functions in body	Synthesis of iodinated thyroid hormones to regulate oxidation within cells affecting temperature, metabolism, nerve and muscle tissue
Storage in body	20-50 mg in the body with one-third stored in the thyroid gland and the remainder in skin, muscles, skeleton and endocrine tissue
Overdose symptoms	More than 2000 mcg/day; Hyperthyroidism, goiter, hyperactivity, hypermetabolism
Deficiency symptoms	Hypothyroidism; myxedema, hypofunction, mental and physical sluggishness
Persons at risk	Thyroiditis, protein malnutrition, pituitary dysfunction, hepatitis
Antagonists	Brussel sprouts, cabbage, cauliflower, peanuts are considered goitergens but

effect inactivated by cooking

Synergists	Thyroid stimulating hormone (TSH)
Comments	Absorbed as inorganic iodide after digestion process and transported in blood as free iodide or protein bound (PBI) TSH causes uptake of iodide by thyroid gland where it becomes part of thyro-globulin complex

ZINC (Zn)

RDA	15 mg/day for male and female
Principle sources	Meats, eggs, seafoods, vegetables
Functions in body	Wound healing and tissue repair Enzyme activity for utilization of vitamin A, transfer of carbon dioxide, production of peptides and protein metabolism, conversion of pyruvic acid to lactic acid, action of insulin
Storage in body	1.4-2.3 Gm in body with 20% in skin and the remaining in bones, teeth, liver, pancreas, brain, prostate, kidneys
Overdose symptoms	More than 2 Gm/day; gastrointestinal irritation, vomiting
Deficiency symptoms	Anorexia, skin changes, impaired wound healing, decreased taste and smell
Persons at risk	Alcoholism, malabsorption syndromes, chronic renal failure, hyperalimentation, living in areas where soil is deficient in zinc
Antagonists	High intake of fiber, calcium and phytate
Synergists	Vitamin A

Comments	40% absorbed in small intestine

COPPER (Cu)

RDA	2.0-3.0 mg/day for male and female
Principle sources	Oyster, nuts, shellfish, liver, kidneys, legumes, raisins
Functions in body	Bone development, formation of hemoglobin, melanin pigment, synthesis of phospholipids, nervous system myelin maintenance, energy production, purine metabilism and fatty acid oxidation, iron metabolism
Storage in body	100-150 mg in body in all tissues with a higher concentration in the liver and brain; eliminated in the feces
Overdose symptoms	More than 250 mg/day; anemia, thyroid dysfunction; hypercupremia
Deficiency symptoms	Hypocupremia, hypothermia, depigmentation of hair and skin, cerebral degeneration, Wilson's disease, bone disease, protein malnutrition
Persons at risk	Use of penicillamine, long term TPN, sprue, malabsorption syndromes and renal diseases, cirrhosis of liver, thyroid dysfunction, leukemias, anemia
Antagonists	Penicillamine
Synergists	Iron, zinc, molybdenum
Comments	Absorbed by stomach and small intestines Majority is bound to protein and small amount to albumin and amino acids; does not exist in free form

MANGANESE (Mn)

RDA	2.5-5.0 mg/day for male and female
Principle sources	Coffee, tea, legumes, whole grains, nuts, fruits and vegetables
Functions in body	Protein and energy metabolism Synthesis of cartilage, prothrombin and gluconeogenesis
Storage in body	12-20 mg in body mostly in liver and kidneys; excreted in feces via the bile
Overdose symptoms	More than 1 Gm/day; neuromuscular disturbances
Deficiency symptoms	Abnormal formation of bone and cartilage, impaired glucose tolerance but none reported in humans
Persons at risk	Poor dietary intake, malnutrition
Antagonists	None known
Synergists	Magnesium
Comments	Absorbed from small intestine but main sites of uptake are the mitochondria

SELENIUM (Se)

RDA	0.05-0.2 mg/day for male and female
Principle sources	Seafood, liver, kidneys
Functions in body	Immune activity, synthesis of ATP, cell protection
Storage in body	Highest concentrations in liver, pancreas, kidneys, pituitary

Excreted in feces

Overdose symptoms	More than 0.4 mcg/day; only shown in animals
Deficiency symptoms	Only shown in animals
Persons at risk	Related to dietary intake of meats and water containing Se
Antagonists	Sulfur
Synergists	None known
Comments	Absorbed in intestines

FLOURIDE (Fl)

RDA	1.5-4.0 mg/day for male and female
Principle source	Drinking water
Functions in body	Bone and teeth structure, prevention of caries
Storage in body	Not stored; excreted in urine
Overdose symptoms	More than 80 mg/day; mottling and discoloration of teeth, increased bone density and calcification; inhibition of enzyme activity in phosphate metabolism
Deficiency symptoms	Osteoporosis, increased dental caries
Persons at risk	Elderly
Antagonists	None
Synergists	Calcium, magnesium, phosphorus
Comments	Absorbed in the intestines

Fluoridation of water decreases dental caries

CHROMIUM

RDA	0.05-0.2 mg/day for male and female
Principle sources	Yeast, meat, cheese, whole grains
Functions in body	Promotes utilization of insulin and maintains glucose tolerance
Storage in body	6 mg in body distributed in all tissues Excreted in urine
Overdose symptoms	More than 500 mg/day
Deficiency symptoms	Hyperglycemia
Persons at risk	Diabetics, elderly, malnutrition
Antagonists	None known
Synergists	Glucose
Comments	Released from tissues with glucose intake; absorbed in the intestines

MOLYBDENUM

RDA	0.15-0.5 mg/day for male and female
Principle sources	Grains, legumes, liver, kdineys
Functions in body	Xanthine, aldehyde and sulfite oxidation; nitrogen fixation in plants
Storage in body	Low concentrations in all parts of the body Eliminated in the feces

Overdose symptoms	More than 1000 mcg/day; goutlike responses
Deficiency symptoms	None known
Persons at risk	Malnutrition
Antagonists	Copper, sulfur
Synergists	None known
Comments	Absorbed in the intestines Content in food depends on con-centration in soil

ELECTROLYTES

Any substance that can dissociate into its component ions in a fluid is an electrolyte. Cations carry a positive charge (+) and anions carry a negative charge (-). In the body solutions, these are equal. They are measured by milliequivalents (mEq). Cations are sodium, calcium, magnesium and potassium; anions are chloride, phosphate, sulfate, bicarbonate and organic acids. The major electrolytes (sodium, chloride and potassium) are covered in this section.

SODIUM (Na⁺)

RDA	1100-3300 mg/day for male and female
Principle sources	Table salt (NaCl), bread, cheeses, whole grains, milk, dried fruit; all foods and additives/perservatives
Functions in body	Regulation of acid-base balance in combination with chloride and bicarbonate Maintains osmotic pressure of fluids Maintains muscle activity and permeability of cells
Storage in body	63 Gm in body; one-third of total found in bones and the remainder in extracellular fluid Excreted in urine, sweat
Overdose symptoms	More than 18 Gm/day or 30 Gm/day as NaCl; hypertension, edema
Deficiency sympotms	Fluid losses, dehydration
Persons at risk	Renal diseases, hypertension, vomiting, diarrhea, Addison's disease
Antagonists	None

Synergists	Chloride, bicarbonate
Comments	Absorbed in the ileum Decreased Na intake causes increased aldosterone secretion and visa-versa

CHLORIDE (Cl⁻)

RDA	1700-5100 mg/day for male and female
Principle sources	Table salt (NaCl)
Functions in body	Regulation of osmotic pressure, fluid balance, acid-base balance, production of hydrochloric acid, assists blood to carry carbon dioxide to lungs and conservation of potassium
Storage in body	85 Gm in body with 15% chloride, most concentrated in cerebrospinal fluid and gastrointestinal secretions and least in muscle and nerve tissue; extracellular fluid anion Excreted in the urine
Overdose symptoms	Same as sodium and occur at same time as for sodium
Deficiency sympotms	Fluid losses, dehydration
Persons at risk	Endocrine disorders, diarrhea, loss of gastric secretions during suction, vomiting, profuse sweating
Antagonists	None
Synergists	Sodium, potassium
Comments	Absorbed in intestines

70

POTASSIUM (K$^+$)

RDA	1875-5625 mg/day for male and female
Principle sources	Chicken, veal, beef, pork, liver, dried fruits, oranges, broccoli, squash
Functions in body	Influence on muscle activity including heart muscle, protein synthesis, maintains acid-base balance and osmotic pressure, contributes to enzyme activity
Storage in body	150 Gm in body with concentration in the intracellular fluid 30 times more than in extracellular fluid Excreted in the urine
Overdose symptoms	More than 12 Gm/day; hyperkalemia, bradycardia, oliguria, paresthesia, tingling and twitching of extremities, abdominal cramps
Deficiency symptoms	Hypokalemia, hypotension, vertigo, nausea, vomiting, diarrhea, muscle weakness, leg cramping, arrhythmias, confusion, depression, irritability
Persons at risk	Diuretic therapy, diarrhea, laxatives, diabetic acidosis, malnutrition
Antagonists	None
Synergists	None
Comments	Absorbed in the intestines Kidneys are major regulatory mechanism for potassium balance

CALCULATION OF CALORIC CONTENT/NEEDS

A general recommendation by the Food and Nutrition Board of the National Research Council is the following:

WOMEN

Age 51-75   1800 calories/day or a reduction of 10% of the mature adult

Age 76 and over   1600 calories/day or a reduction of 20% of the mature adult

MEN

Age 51-75   2400 calories/day or a reduction of 10% of the mature adult

Age 76 and over   2050 calories/day or a reduction of 20% of the mature adult

Energy is measured in kilocalories (kcal). A kcal is a representation of the amount of heat needed to raise 1 kg (1000 Gm) of water 1 degree C. The established energy value for the fuel producing nutrients are:

Protein =   4 kcal/Gm

Carbohydrate =   4 kcal/Gm

Fat =   9 kcal/Gm

If the composition of the food is known, the kcal is calculated as follows:

1 cup whole milk = 9 Gm protein, 12 Gm carbohydrate, 9 Gm fat

$$9 \times 4 = \quad 36$$

$$12 \times 4 = \quad 48$$

$$9 \times 9 = \underline{\quad 81}$$

165 kcal Total

A chart of foods and their contents is used to find the composition amounts of each nutrient in a measured amount of food for calculation of kcal.

To calculate the amount of calories needed by a client, the height, weight and age is used to determine the basal energy expenditure (BEE) which is measured in calories/day.

Height is converted into centimeters (cm) using the equivalency:

1 inch = 2.54 cm, therefore a 5 ft client = 60 in ($5 \times 12 = 60$)

60 in. x 2.54 = 152.4 cm

Weight is converted into kilograms (kg) using the equivalency:

1 kg = 2.2 lb, therefore a 105 lb client = 48.1 kg ($^{105}/_{2.2} = 48.1$)

Formula to calculate BEE for male:

66 + (13.7 x wt. in kg.) + (5 x ht in cm) - (6.8 x age)

Formula to calculate BEE for female:

$$655 + (9.6\ x \text{ wt in kg}) + (1.8\ x \text{ ht in cm}) - (4.7\ x \text{ age})$$

Using the above formula, the calculation for calorie needs for a women of 70 years of age who is 5 ft tall (152.4 cm) and weighs 105 lb (48.1 kg) is:

$$655 + (9.6\ x\ 48.1 \text{ kg}) + (1.8\ x\ 152.4 \text{ cm}) - (4.7\ x\ 70)$$

$$655 + (461.76) + (274.32) - (329)$$

BEE = 1062.08 or 1062 calories/day required for body at rest

Formula to estimate BEE for male:

1 cal/kg/hour

Formula to estimate BEE for female:

0.9 cal/kg/hour

Using the estimated method for the same client:

$$0.9\ x\ 48.1 \text{ kg} = 43.29/\text{hour} \qquad 43.29\ x\ 24 \text{ hour} = 1038.96$$

To calculate an estimate of a desired weight of a client that is either underwieght or overweight, the following formula may be used for a medium framed person:

	Males	Females
1st 5 ft of height	106 lb	100 lb
Added for every additional inch	6 lb	5 lb

10% of total body weight is added for a large framed person

10% of total body weight is subtracted for a small framed person

Using the above formula for a large framed male who is 5 ft 9 in and weighs 170 lb, the calculation for his desired weight is:

Desired wt =	$106 + (9 \times 6)$
	$106 + 54$
Desired wt =	160 lb for medium frame

The adjustment for a large male is 10% of 160 lb or 16 lb

Desired wt =	$160 + 16$
Desired wt=	176 lb

This client is 6 lb overweight

General recommendations by the U.S. Department of Health, Education, and Welfare, Public Health Service for desired weights for men and women of specific heights may be used instead of using the calculation method outlined above.

Height (ft in)	Men Weight (lb)			Women Weight (lb)		
	Average	Acceptable weight		Average	Acceptable weight	
4 10				102	92	119
4 11				104	94	122
5 0				107	96	125
5 1				110	99	128
5 2	123	112	141	113	102	131
5 3	127	115	144	116	105	134
5 4	130	118	148	120	108	138
5 5	133	121	152	123	111	142
5 6	136	124	156	128	114	146
5 7	140	128	161	132	118	150
5 8	145	132	166	136	122	154
5 9	149	136	170	140	126	158
5 10	153	140	174	144	130	163
5 11	158	144	179	148	134	168
6 0	162	148	184	152	138	173
6 1	166	152	189			
6 2	171	156	194			
6 3	176	160	199			
6 4	181	164	204			

Average indicates medium frame

Acceptable range indicates small and large frames

Weight in lb and height in ft and in can be converted to kg and cm if necessary

CALCULATION OF FLUID NEEDS

Total body water decreases with age. In young males, 60% of total body weight is water compared to 52% in the elderly male. In young females, 52% of total body weight is water compared to 46% in the elderly female. The normal adult gains and loses approximately 2400 ml fluids/day and the ratio bewteen the two I&O determines the presence of fluid disturbances. Serious imbalances can occur quickly in the elderly from tube feedings, use of diuretics, laxatives, IV therapy and malnutrition. The average amounts and routes of fluid losses and gains are:

Fluid Losses/Day		Fluid Gains/Day	
800-1500 ml	Urine	1000-1250 ml	Oral liquids
250-350 ml	Stool	650-1250 ml	Foods
100-250 ml	Perspiration	200-400 ml	Metabolic oxidation
250-350 ml	Skin (Insensible)		
350 ml	Lungs		
1900-2800 ml	Total Losses /Day	1850-2900 ml	Total Gains /Day
	Other Losses Tears, vomiting, diarrhea, wound exudate, suction, hemorrhage		Other Gains Tube feedings, parenteral feedings and/or fluids

Usually, weight is used in the calculation of fluid needs for a 24 hour period of time. To calculate the amount of fluid needed by a client:

Allow 100 ml/kg for the first 10 kg body weight

Then add 50 ml/kg for the next 10 kg body weight

After the first 20 kg, add 15 ml/kg body weight

For a 76 kg client:

100 ml x 10 kg = 1000 ml

50 ml x 10 kg = 500 ml

15 ml x 56 kg = 840 ml

2340 ml/day

Another method to estimate fluid needs for 24 hours is:

Allow 1000 ml for every 1000 kcal in 24 hour dietary intake

For a client receiving a 1800 kcal diet:

1000 ml = 1000 kcal

800 ml = 800 kcal

1800 ml.day

Fluids are generally replaced during the day and may be scheduled for administration during shifts if the client is in a long term facility as follows:

7-3 shift	1/2 of total calculated 24 hour fluids
3-11 shift	1/3 of total calculated 24 hour fluids
11-7 shift	1/6 of total calculated 24 hour fluids

This schedule may be modified for an individual client as some elderly may do better with fluid intake spread over day hours taking 100-150 ml/hour and not taking fluids before bedtime or during the night.

To increase fluids for a client, the 24 hour amount would be doubled, but for an elderly client, fluids should be increased slowly over a period of time that would not create a fluid overload. This does not mean, however, that the elderly should not be treated for dehydration as vigorously as any other client.

CHAPTER V
DIETS AND MENUS

CLEAR LIQUID DIET

INDICATIONS
Acute illnesses and infection
Pre-operative
Post-operative
Step #1 from NPO to Regular diet
Temporary food intolerance
Preparation for some laboratory test

RESTRICTIONS
Solid or pureed foods
Milk and milk products
Carbonated/caffeine containing sodas
Fruit juices with pulp

INCLUSIONS
Ginger ale, fruit flavored drinks
Water, coffee, tea
Clear fruit juices, lemonade
Popsicles
Broth, boullion, consommé
Plain gelatin
Hard, clear candies, honey, sugar

COMMENTS
Limited nutritional value; deficient in
protein, minerals, calories, vitamins
Provides fluids and relieves thirst

ADDITIONAL
INTERVENTIONS
Offer fluids frequently; q1-2h
feeding intervals
Provide privacy and avoid exposure to
those having more advanced diet

SAMPLE CLEAR LIQUID DIET

BREAKFAST   Cereal beverage
                   Apple or cranberry juice
                   Coffee, tea and sugar/honey

MID-MORNING   Ginger ale
                   Clear broth

LUNCH   Clear, flavored gelatin
                   Strained fruit juice
                   Tea, coffee and sugar/honey/syrup

MID-AFTERNOON   Popsicle

DINNER   Fruit flavored drink
                   Consommé
                   Plain, clear gelatin
                   Tea, coffee and sugar/honey
                   Clear sugar candy

EVENING   Grape juice

FULL LIQUID DIET

INDICATIONS

Acute gastritis and infections
Step #2 from NPO to Regular diet
Febrile conditions
Intolerance for solid food
Extreme weakness of client

RESTRICTIONS

Solid or pureed foods

INCLUSIONS

All included in Clear Liquid diet
Milk, milk drinks
Non-carbonated beverages
Coffee, tea, decaffeinated coffee
Strained fruit and vegetable juices
Cooked refined cereals/gruel
Custard, pudding, ice cream, sherbet
Gelatin, popsicles
Broth, creamed soups, bouillon
Butter, margarine, cream
Clear, hard candy, sugar, honey

COMMENTS

Inclusions are foods that are liquid at
room temperature
More satisfied feeling after meals than
with Clear Liquid

ADDITIONAL
INTERVENTIONS

Offer 6 feedings/day or 2-4 hour feeding
intervals
Offer fluids frequently
Advance to regular diet as soon as
possible for complete nutritional
requirement intake

SAMPLE FULL LIQUID DIET

BREAKFAST   Strained orange juice
                             Oatmeal gruel with cream
                             Milk or eggnog
                             Coffee, tea, cream and sugar/honey

MID-MORNING   Sherbet

LUNCH   Tomato juice
                             Cream of potato soup
                             Fruit drink
                             Vanilla ice cream
                             Milk, coffee, tea with cream/sugar

MID-AFTERNOON   Flavored yogurt

DINNER   Cranberry juice
                             Cream of chicken soup
                             Pudding
                             Milk, coffee, tea with cream/sugar

EVENING   Hot cocoa or milk shake

LOW RESIDUE/BLAND DIET

INDICATIONS

Indigestion, esophageal reflux
Colitis, irritable bowel, gastritis
Diarrhea
Chemotherapy/Radiation therapy

RESTRICTIONS

Milk and milk products limited
Alcohol, fruit juices with pulp
Raw fruits and vegetables and those with skins
Nuts and seeds; condiments
Rich or spiced gravies, sauces
All fried foods, hot breads
Jams, yogurt with fresh fruit
Coarse cereals and whole grain breads
Smoked, pickled or cured meats
Rich desserts (pies, cakes, cobblers)
Corn, onions, dried beans, peas
Coconut, raisins

INCLUSIONS

All beverages except alcohol
White bread, rolls, crackers
Rice, noodles, macaroni, spaghetti
Cooked cereals, dry cereal without bran
All eggs but fried, cottage, cheddar
and American cheese
Lean, tender, ground, broiled, baked
or stewed meats,canned tuna or
salmon, chicken or turkey without
skin, liver, crisp bacon
Broth, cream and vegetable soups,
bouillon
Butter, margarine, cream, oil, mayonaise
Tender cooked vegetables, vegetable juices
Strained fruit juices, ripe bananas,
applesauce, stewed or canned fruits
without skins
Custards, puddings, sherbet, plain ice
cream, angel food or sponge cake,
plain cookies

Sugar, vinegar, lemon juice, spices as tolerated

COMMENTS
Hot and cold foods should be eaten slowly if at all; foods are generally soft with no high fiber inclusions
Milk products limited to 2 cups daily
Diet reduces amount of fecal material in the lower bowel

ADDITIONAL
INTERVENTIONS
Food tolerances and preferences must have high priority in selections
Offer 6 small meals/day to avoid distention
Evening feeding may be eliminated to reduce acid secretion during night

SAMPLE LOW RESIDUE/BLAND DIET

BREAKFAST   Cranapple juice
                          Cooked oatmeal with cream or milk
                          Scrambled egg
                          Slice white toast with margarine/butter
                          Milk; coffee, tea with cream/sugar

MID-MORNING   Milk shake

LUNCH   Chicken breast, baked
                          White bread, roll
                          Mashed potato
                          Tender asparagus with butter
                          Ripe banana, sugar cookies
                          Milk, tea with cream/sugar

MID-AFTERNOON   Plain yogurt

DINNER   Baked trout
                          Rice, buttered
                          Cooked carrots
                          White bread with margarine/butter
                          Custard
                          Milk, coffee, tea with cream/sugar

EVENING   Applesauce, slice angel food cake

MECHANICAL SOFT DIET

INDICATIONS

Chewing, swallowing difficulties
(neurosensory, neuromuscular)
Poor dentition
Between acute illness and convalescence
Weakness
Gastrointestinal disorders
Chemotherapy/radiation therapy
Step between Liquid-General diet

RESTRICTIONS

All fried foods
All highly spiced foods
High fiber foods; raw fruits/vegetables
Foods with nuts, seeds
Pulpy fruits, prunes, unpeeled fruits

INCLUSIONS

All beverages
White, whole wheat, rye bread without
seeds, saltine or graham crackers
Cooked or prepared refined cereals
Plain cakes, cookies, puddings, custards;
smooth ice cream, sherbet, gelatin,
fruit slushes
Egg, butter, margarine, vegetable oils,
salad dressing, white sauce
All fruit juices, cooked or canned
fruits without skins, ripe banana,
orange/grapefruit sections
Chopped, ground, pureed or tender meats
Cream, cottage, mild cheddar cheese
Casseroles, broth and cream soups and
soups with soft vegetables
Potatoes, hominy, rice, spaghetti,
noodles, macaroni
All vegetable juices, cooked or canned
tender vegetables
Sugar, honey, syrup, clear jelly

COMMENTS	Offer foods with a moist consistency
	Nutritionally adequate diet
	Restrict food preparation and seasoning for individual client
	Avoid any inclusions that give rise to difficulty in chewing, use of facial muscles, swallowing
	Any soft, chopped, ground, pureed foods may be included
	Modification of Light or Soft diet
ADDITIONAL INTERVENTIONS	Offer 6 feedings/day or 3 meals with between meal feedings
	Encourage food in bite-sized amounts at one time
	Allow time; do not rush through meal
	Foods with texture are easier to control in mouth and swallow
	Position upright for meals

SAMPLE MECHANICAL SOFT DIET

BREAKFAST

Orange sections
Farina with milk or cream
Soft cooked egg
Whole wheat toast with butter, jelly
Milk; coffee, tea with cream/sugar

MID-MORNING

Fruit slush

LUNCH

Vegetable soup
Tender roast beef
Baked potato
Buttered spinach
Tomato juice
Slice white bread with margarine/butter
Smooth ice cream
Milk; milk shake

MID-AFTERNOON

Eggnog, yogurt

DINNER

Baked white fish in cream sauce
Tender cooked buttered carrots
Slice whole wheat bread with margarine
Canned pears
Sponge cake slice
Milk; coffee, tea with cream/sugar

EVENING

Plain cookies, pudding

PUREED SOFT/BLENDERIZED DIET

INDICATIONS
Chewing, swallowing difficulties
Tooth pain, loss
Poor fitting dentures
Gastrointestinal impairment
Extreme weakness

RESTRICTIONS
All fried foods
All gas-forming foods
Spicy foods

INCLUSIONS
Milk, milk drinks, egg if not fried
Carbonated beverages, fruit drinks
Coffee, tea, decaffeinated coffee
White toast, saltine, graham crackers
Cooked or prepared refined cereals
Custard, pudding, ice cream, sherbet,
gelatin, popsicles
Plain cake and cookies
Fruit slushes, fruit juices, ripe
banana, vegetable juices
Pureed cooked or canned fruit and
vegetables
Butter, margarine, cream, vegetable oils,
salad dressing, white sauce
Broths and cream soups with pureed
vegetables and meats
Pureed or finely ground beef, lamb,
veal, chicken, turkey, lean pork,
fish in broth or cream sauce
Cream and cottage cheese, mild cheese
Mashed potato, rice, noodles, hominy,
spaghetti (if able to chew)
Honey, sugar, syrup, jelly, clear hard
candy

COMMENTS
Food consistency dependent on appetite,
ability to chew, dysphagia

ADDITIONAL INTERVENTIONS	Offer 6 feedings/day
	Encourage to take small amounts of food at a time
	Allow time; do not rush through meal
	Place in upright position; encourage to participate in communal meals

SAMPLE PUREED/BLENDERIZED DIET

BREAKFAST
Orange juice
Corn flakes or puffed rice with milk
Soft cooked egg
Slice white toast with margarine, jelly
Milk; coffee, tea with cream/sugar

MID-MORNING
Chocolate milk shake

LUNCH
Strained vegetable soup
Ground chicken pattie
Mashed white potato
Pureed carrots
V-8 juice
Slice white bread with margarine/butter
Custard
Milk; coffee, tea with cream/sugar

MID-AFTERNOON
Ice cream or fruit slush

DINNER
Creamed, ground beef sirloin on noodles
Pureed grean beans
Slice white bread with margarine/butter
Pureed peaches with slice angel food cake
Milk; coffee, tea with cream/sugar

EVENING
Eggnog or 2 graham crackers

GENERAL DIET

INDICATIONS
Ambulatory clients
Ability to eat and tolerate any food or
food combinations

RESTRICTIONS
Fried foods, spices and pastries in
moderation
Modifications in prescribed therapeutic
diets

INCLUSIONS
All foods permitted

COMMENTS
Normal, adequate well-balanced diet

ADDITIONAL
INTERVENTIONS
Encourage communal eating
Allow as much time as needed for meals
Provide assistive aids for self feeding
if needed
Assist with eating as needed

SAMPLE GENERAL DIET

BREAKFAST   Grapefruit
Corn flakes with milk or cream
Poached egg on white toast
Butter, margarine, jelly
Milk; coffee, tea with cream/sugar

MID-MORNING   Chocolate milk shake

LUNCH   Beef, vegetable soup
Turkey, tomato, lettuce club sandwich on
white toast with salad dressing
Creamed potatoes
Buttered peas
Gelatin
Milk, carbonated beverage

MID-AFTERNOON   Ice cream, cookies

DINNER   Lamb chop
Sweet potato
Lettuce salad with dressing
Cauliflower
Whole wheat bread with margarine/butter
Angel food cake slice with fruit
Milk; coffee, tea with cream/sugar

EVENING   Fruit, fruit yogurt

HIGH FIBER DIET

INDICATIONS
Constipation, diverticular disease
Prevention of intestinal disorders
Possibly to lower cholesterol levels

RESTRICTIONS
Refined foods and grains

INCLUSIONS
Whole wheat and grain breads, crackers
Bran type cereals, oatmeal, shredded wheat, wheat germ
Wild rice, cornmeal, buckwheat, groats, barley
Fresh fruits with skins; dried fruits
Raw and slightly steamed vegetables
Legumes, nuts, seeds
Oatmeal, bran, raisin muffins/cookies
Popcorn

COMMENTS
High fiber intake will stimulate peristalsis
Promotes bowel evacuation without straining
Prunes contain a laxative agent (dihydroxphenyl isatin)
Dietary fiber refers to all undigestible carbohydrates and lignin from plants

ADDITIONAL
INTERVENTIONS
Increase daily fluid intake to 8-10 glasses/day
Encourage increase in activity
Fiber is usually added to General diet
Recommended daily intake of fiber is 6-10 Gm or 800 Gm fruits and vegetables

SAMPLE HIGH FIBER DIET

BREAKFAST

Grapefruit sections
Raisin all-bran cereal with cream or milk
Poached egg on whole wheat toast
Butter, margarine, jam
Milk; coffee, tea with cream and sugar

MID-MORNING

Apple

LUNCH

Sliced chicken sandwich on whole wheat
with lettuce, tomato, mayonnaise
Chef salad
Oatmeal cookies
Milk; coffee, tea with cream and sugar

MID-AFTERNOON

Banana nut bread slice, dried fruit snack

DINNER

Roast beef
Baked potato with skin
Cole slaw salad
Green beans
Bran muffins with margarine/butter
Strawberries and cream
Milk; coffee, tea with cream and sugar

EVENING

Butter pecan ice cream with raisin
cookies

REDUCED CALORIC/REDUCTION DIET

INDICATIONS

More than 20% over normal weight for height and frame
Maintenance of desired weight

RESTRICTIONS

All fried meats, vegetables
Butter, margarine, oils, creams, gravies
Desserts and sweets; candy, ice cream, cakes, pies, sugar in beverages or foods
Convenience foods

INCLUSIONS

All foods allowed on a General diet with exchanges for low caloric foods in each food group
Low fat dairy products, fat trimmed meats, sugar free foods and beverages
Raw and cooked fruits and vegetables

COMMENTS

Food servings should be reduced
Artificial sweeteners and spices may be used for flavoring
Some fluids are high in calories
Caloric content may be from 1000-1600 calories/day

ADDITIONAL
INTERVENTIONS

Include an exercise program for successful weight loss
Eat regular meals, do not skip meals
Measure portions of foods
Bake, broil or steam foods

SAMPLE REDUCED CALORIC/REDUCTION DIET (1200 CALORIE)

BREAKFAST
1/4 cantaloupe
1 scrambled egg
1 slice whole wheat toast
1 tsp margarine
1/2 cup farina
1 cup low fat milk (skim)
Coffee, tea

LUNCH
1/2 cup tuna (water packed)
2 slices white bread
Lettuce, cucumber, tomato salad
with vinegar
1/2 banana
Coffee, tea or diet soda

DINNER
3 oz baked chicken without skin
1 medium baked potato with 1 tsp
margarine
1/2 cup cooked carrots
Green tossed salad
2 fresh plums
1 cup low fat milk (skim)

SNACK
Fresh apple
Dietetic gelatin

HIGH CALORIC/HIGH PROTEIN DIET

INDICATIONS   Hypermetabolism, chronic wasting
illness, cancer, infections

RESTRICTIONS   No foods restricted
Avoid foods that increase nausea,
vomiting such as greasy foods, foods
with strong odors, rich or sweet
foods, liquids with meals

INCLUSIONS   All foods allowed on a General diet with
exchanges for high caloric and protein
foods in each group
Addition of butter, powdered milk to
sauces, gravies, soups, hot cereals,
eggs, casseroles, rice, potatoes,
pancakes, breads; use milk instead of
water in preparing foods; add meats to
noodles, soups, rice casseroles; add
cheese to noodles, vegetables, soups,
rice, sauces; add mayonnaise or salad
dressing to eggs, sandwiches, salad;
spread peanut butter on bread, cookies,
vegetables, fruit; add nuts to breads,
cookies, cakes, ice cream or as snack;
add honey to toast, cereals, coffee,
tea; add whip cream on desserts; sour
cream or yogurt to vegetables,
dressings, potatoes, gravies

COMMENTS   Food servings should be increased
Anorexia, altered taste and smell
sensations affect food intake
All high caloric and protein foods
should be exchanged for usual foods
eaten

ADDITIONAL INTERVENTIONS	Eat regular meals, do not skip meals
	Serve meals frequently; 4-6/day
	Encourage between meal snacks and high calorie supplemental drinks
	Monitor weight and praise accomplishments

SAMPLE HIGH CALORIC/HIGH PROTEIN DIET

BREAKFAST
Large orange juice
2 poached or scrambled eggs
2 white toast with butter and jelly
Oatmeal with 2 tbsp powdered milk
High protein milk, 1 glass
Coffee, tea with cream and sugar

MID-MORNING
1 can Ensure

LUNCH
Double cheeseburger with lettuce and tomato
Fried potatoes
Fresh peach and grapes
1 glass whole milk or milkshake

MID-AFTERNOON
Fruit and cottage cheese

DINNER
Creamed vegetable soup
Steak
Buttered noodles
Asparagus salad and mayonnaise
Roll and butter
Tapioca pudding with whipped cream
1 glass high protein milk

EVENING
Crackers and peanut butter

IRON RICH DIET

INDICATIONS   Iron deficiency anemia, diseases that
                            interfere with iron absorption

RESTRICTIONS   No foods are restricted

INCLUSIONS   Beef liver, liverwurst, beef
                            Shrimp, dried beans, oatmeal, farina
                            Prunes, raisins, bran flakes, dates
                            Chicken, frankfurter
                            Spinach, peas, potato
                            White, whole wheat bread

COMMENTS   Iron is needed for synthesis of hemoglobin
                            Most iron is supplied by the meat group
                            followed by the bread and cereal group
                            Foods containing ascorbic acid should
                            be encouraged to assist in the
                            absorption of iron

ADDITIONAL   Foods may be selected from General diet
INTERVENTIONS   menus

SAMPLE IRON RICH DIET

BREAKFAST   Stewed prunes
                   Oatmeal
                   White toast and butter or margarine
                   Poached egg or omelet
                   Milk
                   Coffee, tea with cream and sugar

MID-MORNING   Whole orange

LUNCH   Liverwurst on 2 slices bread
                   Tossed salad with dressing
                   Carbonated drink
                   Canned pineapple

MID-AFTERNOON   Raisins, dried fruit

DINNER   Beef liver with onions/bacon
                   Baked potato with butter/sour cream
                   Spinach salad with dressing
                   Buttered peas
                   Whole wheat bread
                   Strawberry cake
                   Coffee, tea with cream and sugar

EVENING   Cookies, custard

PROTEIN RESTRICTED DIET

INDICATIONS   Renal failure, hepatic failure

RESTRICTIONS   Protein foods, mainly meats, eggs and
                       milk products
                       Protein may be restricted to 20 Gm/day
                       and may progress to 40-60 Gm/day
                       Fats and Na, K, P may also be restricted
                       with low protein

INCLUSIONS   Foods low in protein with protein from
                       high biological value sources
                       Foods high in caloric value
                       Carrots, lettuce, onions, radishes, egg-
                       plant, cabbage, squash, cucumbers, tomato
                       Synthetic juices, carbonated drinks
                       Hard candies, coffee, tea
                       Apples, berries, cherries, grapefruit,
                       peaches, pears, pineapple,
                       prunes
                       Butter, margarine, sour cream, oil

COMMENTS   Protein amount should be specified as
                       20 Gm, 40 Gm, 60 Gm and if other
                       restrictions should be enforced
                       High or sufficient calories and
                       nutrients should be provided
                       Protein increases may be in 10 Gm
                       increments as tolerated
                       Multi-vitamins are often prescribed
                       Protein is essential to health and
                       cannot be eliminated for long
                       period of time
                       Compliance is difficult but necessary
                       to reduce workload of kidneys and
                       amount of protein by-products

106

ADDITIONAL
INTERVENTIONS

Consider possibility of other restrictions

Dietary control is an important aspect of dialysis treatment

Milk and eggs are primary sources of essential amino acids for diet inclusion of protein

SAMPLE PROTEIN RESTRICTED DIET

BREAKFAST
2 oz Grape juice
Corn flakes
1 Soft boiled egg
* 2 tsp Butter or margarine
1/4 cup Milk
Coffee, tea with cream and sugar

MID-MORNING
Low protein cookies

LUNCH
* 1/4 cup Tuna
2 Bread slices
* 2 T Mayonnaise
Green salad with lemon or vinegar
Gelatin with whipped topping
Carbonated drink

MID-AFTERNOON
Hard candy or Jelly beans

DINNER
1 oz Baked fish
1/2 cup Mashed potatoes
* Peas with 1 tsp butter
Fruit cocktail
1/2 cup Fruit drink
Coffee, tea with cream and sugar

EVENING
Low protein toast with butter

* Salt-free foods should be used where applicable for renal failure and liver failure.

LOW FAT/CHOLESTEROL DIET

INDICATIONS
Gallbladder, liver or pancreatic diseases
Cardiovascular diseases
Prevention of atherosclerosis

RESTRICTIONS
All fried and fatty foods
Avocados, olives, nuts
Cheeses, whole milk, ice cream
Organ meats, skin of chicken, fatty meats, shrimp
Sauces and gravies and creams
Butter, lard, high saturated oil
Cakes, pastries containing egg
No more than 3 eggs/week

INCLUSIONS
Lean meats, chicken, fish that is baked, broiled, steamed
Cholesterol-free oils, margarine, dressings within fat restriction
All fruits and vegetables prepared and served without butter, toppings
Skim milk, low fat/cholesterol cheese and yogurt, egg whites
All breads. cakes made with minimal eggs and whole milk
Legumes and nuts
Pasta products without eggs

COMMENTS
Low fat diet reduces gallbladder contractions and pain
Fat is not added in cooking foods
Seasonings will improve taste of food
Fat content is modified to increase ratio of polyunsaturated fatty acids to saturated fatty acids
Calories should be modified if combined with a reduction diet

ADDITIONAL
INTERVENTIONS

Diet may be low fat or low cholesterol
and low saturated fat depending on
underlying factors

Many cholesterol-free products on the
market to choose from

SAMPLE LOW FAT/CHOLESTEROL DIET

BREAKFAST

Orange juice
Farina
Low cholesterol scarmbled egg
Slice toast with margarine
Skim milk
Coffee, tea with sugar or sweetener

LUNCH

Skinless baked chicken
Mashed potato with margarine
Green salad with tomato and low
fat/cholesterol dressing
Slice bread
Angel food cake slice
Iced tea, coffee with sugar

DINNER

Lean hamburger pattie
Hamburger bun
Green beans with seasoning
Rice with margarine/tomato sauce
Peach and low cholesterol cottage
cheese salad
Watermelon
Skim milk

SNACKS

Whole apple
Pudding made with skim milk

LOW SODIUM DIET

INDICATIONS   Renal diseases, fluid retention
Hypertension, heart failure

RESTRICTIONS   Commercially prepared foods made with
milk and milk products
Canned vegetables, juices, frozen products
processed with salt
Potato chips, snack foods, sauerkraut
Crystallized or glazed fruit, dried
fruit with sodium sulfite added
Breads or commercial mixes made with
salt, MSG, baking soda or powder
Cereals, crackers except low sodium
Canned, smoked, salted meats, cold cuts,
tongue, fish, anchovies, herring
Shellfish, salted butter, margarine,
bacon, commercial salad dressings
unless low salt, salted nuts
Pudding, beverage, cake, cookie and
other types of mixes
Pickles, olives, relish, soy sauce

INCLUSIONS   Skim and whole fresh milk
Fresh, frozen or canned fruits and
vegetables without sodium
Low sodium breads, cereals, crackers
Meat, poultry, fish, eggs, low sodium
cheese and peanut butter
Unsalted butter, margarine, cooking
oils, and fats
Low salt beverages, candies, gelatin,
jams and jellies, syrup

COMMENTS   Totally salt free diet impossible as
sodium is found in most foods
Some sodium is essential for life
Restriction should be specific:
Mild: 2500-4500 mg/day

112

Moderate: 1000-2000 mg/day
Strict: 500 mg/day
Severe: 250 mg/day
1 mEq Na = 23 mg

ADDITIONAL
INTERVENTIONS

Salt or seasonings containing sodium is
not added when preparing foods

Remove salt shaker from table or tray
and add none to prepared food

Limit milk products to 2 cups/day

Modify sodium allowance by restricting
milk products and meat and using salt
free foods as needed

Use salt substitutes when possible

Avoid use of low salt, salt free or
salt poor unless desired level of
salt included

Provide information about medications
that include sodium (aspirin, ant-
acids, laxatives, cough syrups)

Instruct to read all food labels for
amount of sodium

SAMPLE LOW SODIUM DIET

BREAKFAT
* 1/2 cup puffed wheat
1 cup milk
* Slice toast and margarine
Poached egg
Coffee, tea with sugar

LUNCH
* Chicken salad sandwich with mayonnaise
Green salad
Fresh apple
1/2 cup sherbert
Iced tea, coffee

DINNER
Moderate portion roast beef
Medium sized baked potato
* Margarine or 1 tbsp sour cream
1/2 cup beets
1 roll
* 1 cup pudding
Coffee, tea with sugar

Use salt free foods

DIABETIC DIET

INDICATIONS   Diabetes mellitus (IDDM, NIDDM)

RESTRICTIONS   All concentrated sweets, sugar, candy,
                         honey, cakes, cookies, pies, sodas
                         Sautrated fats, meats, oils, butter,
                         whole milk products
                         Brown sugar, powdered sugar, jams,
                         jellies, molasses, syrups
                         Commerically prepared foods made with
                         sugar; canned fruits, drinks

INCLUSIONS   Skim or low fat milk and milk products
                         Unflavored yogurt
                         All fresh, frozen and canned vegetables
                         except those in sauces or butter
                         Legumes, corn, lima beans, potatoes
                         Peas, pumpkin, squash
                         All fresh fruits, canned fruit without
                         sugar, frozen fruits without sugar
                         All breads and cereals except quick
                         breads or sweat rolls, coffee cake,
                         doughnuts
                         Biscuit, cornbread, crackers, muffin,
                         pancake, waffle
                         All meats of a proper amount
                         Animal and vegetable fats
                         Noodles, spaghetti, macaroni
                         Spices, herbs, lemon, vinegar

COMMENTS   Measure and eat foods in the correct
                         portions stated on exchange lists
                         Eat regular meals, do not skip meals
                         Use polyunsaturated fats
                         Calories should maintain ideal body
                         weight
                         Balance diet with exercise and insulin

ADDITIONAL INTERVENTIONS	Artificial sweeteners may be used
	Maintain regular exercise program
	Lists are available from commercial food companies, fast food restaurants for food composition
	Snack may supplement diet and should contain sufficient carbohydrate to maintain glucose in normal range until time for next meal
	If on insulin, notify physician for adjustments during an illness
	Exchange selections should reflect allowable caloric intake as well as protein, carbohydrate, fat content

SAMPLE DIABETIC DIET

BREAKFAST
1/2 cup Orange juice
1 cup Corn flakes
1/2 cup Low fat milk
Scrambled egg
Slice toast with margarine
Coffee, tea with sweetener

LUNCH
3 oz Hamburger
Hamburger bun
Green tossed salad with 2 tbsp dressing
1/2 cup Low fat milk
Apple
Diet soda

MID-AFTERNOON
4 Crackers and 1 oz cheese

DINNER
3 oz Broiled chicken
1/2 cup Mashed potato
Small dinner roll with margarine
1 cup Green beans
1 cup Low fat milk
1/2 cup Canned water packed pears
Coffee, tea with sweetener

EVENING
1/2 cup Low fat milk
Small orange

HIGH POTASSIUM DIET

INDICATIONS	Potassium loss with use of diuretic
RESTRICTIONS	No restrictions
INCLUSIONS	All fruits especially citrus fruits Bananas, dates, raisins, prunes, melons All vegetables especially broccoli, potatoes, legumes, brussel sprouts, parsnips, rhubarb Whole grain breads, bran cereals, nuts Meat, chocolate, molasses, wheat germ Broth, boullion
COMMENTS	Potassium replacement may be necessary if level too low High potassium foods also contain sodium and should be regulated if on low sodium diet Hypokalemia is the result of K losses of fluids
ADDED INTERVENTIONS	Inform of signs and symptoms of hypokalemia: tingling in extremities, muscle twitching, tetany Increase in dietary intake of potassium depends on type of diuretic (potassium-sparing diuretic)

SAMPLE HIGH POTASSIUM DIET

BREAKFAST
Glass orange juice
Fried egg
Toast with butter, margarine, jelly
Bran cereal
Milk
Coffee, tea with cream and sugar

LUNCH
Tuna salad sandwich on whole grain bread
Lettuce salad with dressing
Banana
Glass milk

DINNER
Meat loaf and gravy
Baked potato with sour cream
Broccoli
Mixed salad with tomato and dressing
Bran muffin
Fresh fruit compote
Coffee, tea with cream and sugar

EVENING
Hot cocoa made with milk
Honeydew, watermelon

POTASSIUM RESTRICTED DIET

INDICATIONS	Renal diseases, renal failure
RESTRICTIONS	Banana, cantaloupe, grapefurit or orange juice, nectarine, potatoes, tomato juice, peaches, watermelon, prunes, figs, dates, avocado, pear Artichokes, asparagus, beets, broccoli, carrots, collard, rutabaga, squash, legumes; skim milk, coffee, tea Soybeans, peanuts, raisins, wheat germ
INCLUSIONS	Lettuce, radishes, tomatoes, green pepper, green beans Cranberry juice and sauce, lemons, blueberries Breads, spaghetti, cottage cheese, eggs, chicken, meats, fish, butter, fats and oils Canned foods that are drained Cornstarch, wheat starch, tapioca
COMMENTS	Restriction ranges from 1500-3000 mg/day with a normal range of intake about 2000-6000 mg (5 mEq = 200 mg) Most foods that contain potassium also contain sodium Amount of restriction should be specific in ordered diet Diet is often combined with sodium and protein restricted diet Hyperkalemia is the result of kidneys inability to excrete potassium
ADDITIONAL INTERVENTIONS	Inform of signs and symptoms of hyperkalemia: nausea, diarrhea, muscle spasms, weakness, irregular pulse Inform to read labels for sodium content

SAMPLE POTASSIUM RESTRICTED DIET

BREAKFAST
Cranberry juice cocktail
Slice bread with butter, margarine
Poached egg
Purffed rice
Milk
Coffee, tea with sugar

LUNCH
Sliced chicken sandwich on white bread
Green salad with lemon
Tapioca
Carbonated drink

DINNER
Meatballs and buttered noodles
Green beans
Cottage cheese and drained pineapple
salad
Lettuce salad with dressing
Baked apple
White dinner roll
Coffee, tea with sugar

CHAPTER VI
EXCHANGE LISTS

FOOD GROUP EXCHANGE LISTS

Exchange lists are used for meal planning to modify diets for those that require special considerations or preferences because of disease or disabling disorders. Groups are divided according to the amount of protein, carbohydrate, fat and calories the food contains. The choices on the lists are about equal and one food may be exchanged for another on the list in planning a complete diet.

Approximate composition of a serving of each nutrient is:

Food	Protein (Gm)	Carbohydrate (Gm)	Fat (Gm)	Calories
Starch/Bread	2	15	trace	70
Meat				
Lean	7	0	3	55
Medium fat	7	0	5	75
High fat	7	0	8	100
Vegetable	2	5	0	25
Fruit	0	10	0	40
Milk				
Skim	8	12	trace	90
Low fat	8	12	5	120
Whole	8	12	8	150
Fat	0	0	5	45

MILK EXCHANGES

12 Gm carbohydrate, 8 Gm protein, trace to 8 Gm fat and 90-150 calories/exchange depending on type of milk

NONFAT MILK:

Skim or nonfat milk	1 cup
Powdered nonfat milk	1/3 cup
Canned evaporated skim milk	1/2 cup
Buttermilk from skim milk	1 cup
Yogurt from skim milk (plain)	1 cup

LOW FAT MILK:

1% or 2% fortified milk	1 cup
Yogurt from 2% milk	1 cup

WHOLE MILK

4% whole milk	1 cup
Canned evaporated milk	1/2 cup
Buttermilk or yogurt (plain) from whole milk	1 cup

CONDITIONS USING THIS MODIFICATION:

Inclusion-   Diabetes mellitus, Malnutrition, Oral deterioration and disorders; High protein/high caloric diet, Full liquid diet, Low residue/bland diet, Mechanical soft/pureed diet, General diet

Exclusion-   Chronic renal failure, Atherosclerosis; Protein restricted diet, Low fat/cholesterol diet, reduced caloric/reduction diet, Clear liquid diet

VEGETABLE EXCHANGES

5 Gm carbohydrate, 2 Gm protein and 25 calories/exchange

Asparagus	1/2 cup
Bean sprouts	1/2 cup
Beets	1/2 cup
Broccoli	1/2 cup
Cabbage or Brussel sprouts	1/2 cup
Carrots	1/2 cup
Cauliflower	1/2 cup
Celery	1/2 cup
Eggplant	1/2 cup
Green pepper	1/2 cup
Beet, chard, collard, kale, mustard, spinach, turnip, dandelion greens	1/2 cup
Mushrooms	1/2 cup
Onions	1/2 cup
Okra, rutabaga, zucchini	1/2 cup
Rhubarb	1/2 cup
Sauerkraut	1/2 cup
Green, yellow string beans	1/2 cup

RAW VEGETABLES USED AS DESIRED:

Lettuce, endive, escarole
Parsely, watercress
Radishes, chinese cabbage

CONDITIONS USING THIS MODIFICATION:

Inclusion-   Diabetes mellitus, Constipation, Diverticular disease; General diet, High fiber diet, High potassium diet, Low fat/cholesterol diet, Reduced caloric/reduction diet

Exclusion -   Bowel inflammatory disease, Oral deterioration and disorders, Diarrhea; Clear and Full liquid diets, Low residue/bland diet, Mechanical soft diet unless pureed, Potassium restricted diet

FRUIT EXCHANGES

10 Gm carbohydrate and 40 calories/exchange

Apple, orange, pear, nectarine	1 small
Apple, pineapple juice, cider	1/3 cup
Applesauce (unsweetened)	1/2 cup
Banana, mango	1/2 small
Apricots, plums, prunes	2 medium
Cherries	10 large
Grapes	12
Blackberries, blueberries, raspberries, pineapple	1/2 cup
Orange, grapefruit juice	1/2 cup
Prune, grape juice	1/4 cup
Dates	2
Peach, persimmon, tangerine	1 medium
Raisins	2 tbsp
Figs (fresh or dried)	1
Strawberries, papaya	3/4 cup
Watermelon	1 cup
Cantaloupe	1/4 small
Honeydew	1/8 medium
Cranberries (unsweetened)	As desired

CONDITIONS USING THIS MODIFICATION:

Inclusion: Diabetes mellitus, Constipation, Diverticular disease; General diet, High fiber diet, High potassium diet, Low fat/cholesterol diet, Reduced caloric/reduction diet

Exclusion: Gastrointestinal inflammatory disorders, Diarrhea; Clear and Full liquid diets, Low residue/bland diet, Mechanical soft except for soft fruits and juices, Potassium restricted diet

BREAD EXCHANGES

15 Gm carbohydrate, 2 Gm protein and 70 calories/exchange

BREAD:

White, whole wheat, rye, pumpernickel, raisin	1 slice
Bagel, English muffin, hamburger or hotdog bun	1/2
Plain roll	1
Bread crumbs	1 tbsp
Tortilla, pita	1

CEREAL:

Cooked cereal, grits, rice, barley, pasta	1/2 cup
Dry bran flakes	1/2 cup
Puffed cereal (unfrosted)	1 cup
Ready-to-eat dry cereals	3/4 cup
Popcorn (plain)	3 cups
Wheat germ	1/4 cup
Flour	2 1/2 tbsp
Cornmeal	2 tbsp

CRACKERS:

Arrowroot	3
Graham	2
Matzo	1/2
Oyster	20
Rye wafer	3
Saltines	6
Soda	4

LEGUMES:

Beans, peas, lentils (dried and cooked)	1/2 cup
Baked beans (canned, no pork)	1/4 cup

STARCHY VEGETABLES:

Corn	1/3 cup
Corn on cob	1 small
Lima beans, green peas, mashed potato, winter squash	1/2 cup
Parsnips	2/3 cup
White potato	1 small
Pumpkin	3/4 cup
Sweet potato, yam	1/4 cup

PREPARED FOODS:

Biscuit	1
Cornbread, cornbread muffin	1
Muffin	1 small
Pancake	1
Waffle	1
Potato or corn chips	15
French fried potatoes	8

CONDITIONS USING THIS MODIFICATION:

Inclusion -   Diabetes mellitus, All condtions with adjustments made for oral disorders, Malnutrition; General diet, High caloric diet

Exclusion -   Those foods with high fat, cholesterol, sodium content, Clear and Full liquid diets, Reduced calorie/reduction diet, Soft/low residue/bland diets except for toast and cooked cereals

MEAT EXCHANGES

LEAN MEATS

7 Gm protein, 3 Gm fat and 55 calories/exchange

Beef (baby beef, chuck, flank, tenderloin, round,   1 oz tripe, ribs, rump)

Lamb (leg, rib, sirloin, chops, roast, shank, shoulder)	1 oz
Pork (rump, shank, ham)	
Veal (loin, rib, cutlets, shoulder, chops)	1 oz
Poultry (chicken, turkey, pheasant, without skin)	1 oz
Fish (fresh or frozen)	1 oz
Canned tuna, salmon, crab, lobster	1/4 cup
Shrimp, scallops, clams, oysters	1 oz
Drained sardines	3
Cottage cheese (dry or 2%)	1/4 cup
Dried beans or peas	1/2 cup
Cheese with less than 5% butterfat	1 oz

MEDIUM FAT MEATS

7 Gm protein, 5 Gm fat and 75 calories/exchange

Beef (ground - 15% fat, round), canned corned beef, rib eye	1 oz
Pork (loin, tenderloin, shoulder arm, or blade, broiled ham, Canadian bacon)	1 oz
Liver, heart, kidney, sweetbreads	1 oz
Creamed cottage cheese	1/4 cup
Cheese (ricotta, farmer's, parmesan, mozzarella)	1 oz
Egg	1
Peanut butter	2 tbsp

HIGH FAT MEATS

7 Gm protein, 8 Gm fat and 100 calories/exchange

Beef (brisket, corned beef, ground beef (chuck), roasts, steaks)	1 oz
Lamb breast, veal breast	1 oz
Pork (spare ribs, loin, ground, country ham	1 oz
Poultry (capon, duck, goose)	1 oz
Cheese (cheddar)	1 oz
Cold cuts	1 slice
Frankfurter	1 small

CONDITIONS USING THIS MODIFICATION:

Inclusion -   Diabetes mellitus, anemia, All conditions with adjustments made for oral disorders, General diet, High protein/caloric diet, Iron rich diet

Exclusions -   Chronic renal failure, Athersclerosis; Clear and full liquid diets, Mechanical soft/low residue/bland diets unless meat pureed, Low protein/reduced caloric diet, low fat/cholesterol, sodium diets unless modified

FAT EXCHANGES

POLYUNSATURATED:
5 Gm fat and 45 calories/exchange

Margarine (corn, soy, safflower, cottonseed, sunflower	1 tsp
Oil (corn, olive, peanut, soy, sunflower, safflower)	1 tsp
Avocado	1/8
Olives	5 small
Pecans	2 large
Walnuts	6 small
Almonds	10 whole
Spanish peanuts	20 whole
Virginia peanuts	10 whole

SATURATED:

Margarine (regular)	1 tsp
Butter	1 tsp
Light cream	1 tbsp
Sour cream	1 tbsp
Heavy cream	1 tbsp
Bacon fat	1 tsp
Crisp bacon	1 strip
French, Italian dressing	1 tbsp
Mayonnaise	1 tsp
Mayonnaise-type salad dressing	2 tsp
Lard	1 tsp
Salt pork	3/4 in cube

CONDITIONS USING THIS MODIFICATION:

Inclusion -   Diabetes mellitus

Exclusion -   Weight reduction, Hypertension,
Coronary artery disease, Athersclerosis,
Cholecystitis/cholelithiasis, Absorption disorders

EXCHANGE LIST FOR HIGH SODIUM FOODS

DIARY PRODUCTS
Regular cheeses
Puddings made from mixes
Commercial buttermilk

BREADS/CEREALS
Commercial granola
Instant cooked cereals
Processed bran type cereals
Saltine crackers, pancake, waffle mixes, Bisquick, pretzels
Baking powder biscuits, muffins
Cornbread, nutbread
Rice or noodle mixed

VEGETABLES
Sauerkraut
Frozen processed with sodium
Tomato, V-8 juices; drink mixes
Creamed or seasoned sauces on vegetables
Potato chips, french fries, instant potatoes

MEAT
Smoked or cured meats (bacon, ham, sausage, hot dogs, cold cuts)
Shellfish, sardines, herring, anchovies, caviar
Canned tuna, salmon, mackerel
Bouillon cubes or dehydrated soups

FATS
Bacon
Salad dressings, mayonnaise
Commercial dips
Salted nuts or seeds

MISCELLANEOUS
Seasonings (salt, baking powder or soda, commerical celery, onion, garlic salts and other seasonings and pepper)
Meat tenderizers, MSG, soy sauce, Worcestershire, horseradish, mustard, chili sauce, steak sauce, barbeque sauce

Olives, pickles, salted popcorn
Commercially prepared frozen or canned dinners, entrees, vegetables
Commercially baked desserts, pastry and cake mixes
Bottled, canned sodas, soft drinks

CONDITIONS USING THIS MODIFICATION:

> Restricted in chronic renal failure and
> cardiovascular disease

EXCHANGE LIST FOR LOW
FAT/CHOLESTEROL FOODS

DIARY PRODUCTS
Skim milk, buttermilk
Cottage cheese, rinsed cheeses with less than 11% fat
Egg whites, cholesterol free egg substitutes
Margarine

BREAD/CEREALS
Enriched white and whole grain breads
English muffins, melba toast
Pita, tortillas
Low fat crackers, graham, matzo, saltine, soda
Hot breads, pancakes, waffles made with substitute egg
All cereals except granola, those with coconut or high fat content

VEGETABLES
All vegetable prepared without butter, cream sauces
Vegetable oils (corn, soy, cottonseed, safflower, peanut)
All vegetable juices

FRUITS
All fruits and fruit juices

MEATS
Lean beef, pork, veal, lamb, (all trimmed of fat before cooking)
Chicken and turkey with skin removed

Low fat, dried cold cuts
Fish, clams, scallops, lobster, oysters
Water packed tuna, salmon
Broth base canned or homemade soups

DESSERTS
Gelatin, ices, low-fat frozen desserts, sherbet
Angel food cake, ginger snaps, vanilla wafers
Pudding made with skim milk, canned fruit

MISCELLANEOUS
Peanut butter, nuts, olives (limited)
Pasta products
Mustard, catsup, steak sauces, gravy made with fat-free broth
Hard candy, gum drops, syrups, honey, jam, jelly, marshmallows
Salad dressings, commercial or homemade, cholesterol-free or made with polyunsaturated fat
Carbonated beverages, cocoa with skim milk

CONDITIONS USING THIS MODIFICATION:
Cardiovascular diseases, Cholecystitis, Obesity

EXCHANGE LIST FOR HIGH POTASSIUM FOODS

FRUITS
Orange, grapefruit, pineapple, whole or juice
Pear, apricot, peach, nectarine (fresh)
Banana, papaya, tangerine
Figs, prunes, dates, raisins
Avocado
Cantaloupe, honeydew melon

VEGETABLES
Broccoli, brussel sprouts
Rutabagas, parsnips
Potatoe, yams
Tomato, whole or juice
Pinto beans
Rhubarb, artichokes
Pumpkin, winter squash

Vegetable juice

MISCELLANEOUS
Pecans, walnuts, peanuts

Molasses

Chocolate, cocoa

CONDITIONS USING THIS MODIFICATION:
Diuretic therapy, Vomiting,
Diarrhea, Restricted in chronic renal failure

EXCHANGE LIST FOR HIGH PROTEIN FOODS

DAIRY PRODUCTS
Milk and milk products
Cheeses and cottage cheese
Brewer's yeast
Egg

VEGETABLES
Lentils
Soybeans

BREAD/CEREALS
Rice
Whole wheat bread

MEAT
Poultry, beef, fish, veal, pork, lamb

MISCELLANEOUS
Peanut butter
Peanuts, sunflower seeds, sesame seeds

CONDITIONS USING THIS MODIFICATIONS:
                    Restricted in chronic renal failure;
                    Useful in Malnutrition

EXCHANGE LIST FOR HIGH FIBER FOODS

FRUITS
Dried fruits (apricots, figs, prunes, dates, pears, raisins)

Raw with skins (apples, plums, peaches, grapes, pears, berries, cherries)

Peeled (oranges, grapefruit, rhubarb)

Canned (grapefruit, mandarin oranges, strawberries)

VEGETABLES
Raw (lettuce, carrots, celery, spinach, cabbage, broccoli, asparagus, cauliflower, corn, peppers, peas, beans, beets)

French fried potatoes and potato chips

NUTS
Peanuts, pecans, brazil, almonds

Popcorn, seeds

BREADS AND CEREALS
Flour and bread (whole wheat, bran, white, cornmeal, buckwheat)

Cereals (All-Bran, Grapenuts, cornflakes, puffed rice or wheat, Rice Krispies, shredded wheat, Special K)

Cookies (oatmeal, dried fruit)

Rice (brown and white)

CONDITIONS USING THIS MODIFICATION:
Constipation, Fecal impaction, Diverticular disease, Heart conditions, Colorectal cancer

EXCHANGE LIST FOR HIGH CALCIUM FOODS

DIARY PRODUCTS
Whole, skim milk
Buttermilk
Eggnog
Half and half
Evaporated canned milk
Cheddar, creamed cottage, American, mozzarella, Swiss, parmesan cheeses
Ice cream
Yogurt
Custard

VEGETABLES
Spinach, broccoli
Collard, turnip, mustard greens
Bok choy, kale
Bean curd (tofu)

NUTS
Almonds, hazelnuts

SEAFOOD
Sardines
Shrimp
Oysters
Salmon

CONDITIONS USING THIS MODIFICATION:
Osteoporosis, Menopause

EXCHANGE LIST FOR HIGH IRON FOODS

BREAD/CEREAL
Oatmeal
Bran flakes
White enriched, whole wheat bread

VEGETABLES
Spinach
Peas, snap beans
Split peas
Potato

MEAT
Liver, beef, liverwurst
Beef patty
Shrimp
Chicken
Frankfurter

FRUIT
Orange
Prunes, raisins

CONDITIONS USING THIS MODIFICATION:
Anemia

CULTURAL/ETHNIC ASPECTS OF EXCHANGES

Listed are limited selections of cultural/ethnic preferences but many other foods are acceptable to these groups especially if they are American born and have become acculturated. The lists are by no means complete and menu planning should be based on a nutritional assessment and exchanges made according to likes and dislikes.

MEXICAN-AMERICAN SELECTIONS

Diary products:	Custard (flan), Monterey jack cheese, rice pudding, milk with chocolate
Fruits and vegetables:	Corn, carrots, chili peppers, tomatoes, prickly pear cactus leaf, wild greens, shredded lettuce; prickly pear cactus fruit, melons, zapote, avocado
Meat, fish, eggs, legumes, nuts:	Pork and pork intestine, goat, tripe, sausage, pinto, garbonzo, calico beans, refried beans, peanuts, eggs, chicken, beef, lamb
Bread, cereals, grains, pasta, rice:	Tortillas, rice, pasta, sweet bread, cornmeal gruel, polvillo, sopapilla
Supplementary:	Salt pork, tequila, lard, guacomole, chili sauce, chili powder, salsa, coriander, cumin, saffron

BLACK-AMERICAN SELECTIONS

Diary products:	Whole, dry or evaporated milk, cottage and cheddar cheese
Fruits and vegetables:	Okra, collard, kale, turnip, mustard greens, beans, onions, sweet potatoes, yams; melons, tangerines
Meat, fish, eggs, legumes, nuts:	Pork and ham, hog jowls, ham hocks, hog maw, fatback, bacon, sausage, heart, lungs, kidneys, brains, pig's feet, tails, ears and snout, neck bones, tongue, spareribs, squirrel, rabbit, opossum, quail, catfish, perch, salted fish, sardines, scallops, crayfish; blackeyed peas, peanuts, pinto and red

	kidney beans
Bread, cereals, grains, pasta, rice:	Hominy grits, biscuits, cornbread, hush puppies, spoon bread, past, baked sweet desserts
Supplementary:	Lard, gravies, molasses, syrups, jams and jellies

ASIAN (CHINESE/JAPANESE) SELECTIONS

Diary products:	Milk, cheese
Fruits and vegetables:	Bamboo shoots, green and yellow beans, bean sprouts, bok choy, eggplant, kale, collard, mustard, radish greens, leeks, mushrooms, peppers, scallions, snow peas, taro, tomatoes, water chestnuts, white radishes; dates, figs, grapes, kumquats, litchee nuts, mangoes, papayas, persimmons, napa cabbage, seaweed, limes, cherries, pomegranates, pickled plums, tangerines
Meat, fish, eggs, legumes, nuts;	Pork, beef, organ meats, goat, duck, carp, oyster, lobster, crab, mackerel, sardines, abalone, eels, squid, octopus, fish sausage, globefish, soybean curd, soybean paste, soybeans, lima and red beans, chestnuts, almonds, cashews
Bread, cereals, grains, pasta, rice:	Rice, noodles, barley, millet, oatmeal
Supplementary:	Soy sauce, sweet and sour sauce, ginger, pickled vegetables, suet, saki, plum sauce, peanut oil, lard, mustard sauce

ITALIAN SELECTIONS

Diary products:	Milk, parmesan, ricotta, romano, provolone and other cheeses, custard
Fruits and vegetables:	Escarole, zucchini, squashes, eggplant, artichokes, peppers, tomatoes, swiss chard, dandelion, mustard greens; fennel, tangerines, figs, persimmons, pomegranates, olives, melons, quinces, dates
Meat, fish, eggs,	Beef, veal, organ meats, lamb, pork,

legumes, nuts:	salami, peppered sausage, prosciutto, sardines, anchovies, shellfish, octopus, snails, squid; chick peas, lentils, almonds, pistachios, walnuts, chestnuts
Bread, cereals, grains, pasta, rice:	White Italian bread, all pasta products, pizza filled pastries
Supplementary:	Olive oil, garlic, vinegar, oregano, basil, saffron, parsley, salt pork, espresso, lard, wines

MIDEASTERN SELECTIONS

Diary products:	Soured milk (cow, goat, sheep), soft and hard cheeses, yogurt
Fruits andvegetables:	Onions, tomatoes, okra, peppers, eggplant, cucumbers, grape leaves, artichoke, cabbage, leeks, greens; olives, melons, dates, figs, grapes, quinces, apricots, plums, currants, raisins, prunes, cherries, oranges
Meat, fish, eggs, legumes, nuts:	Mutton, lamb, goat, beef and pork, camel, goose, duck, salted and smoked fish, eggs; lentils, chick peas, soybeans, peanuts, pistachios, caraway and sesame seeds
Bread,cereals,grains, pasta, rice:	Dark and whole creacked wheat bread, rice, barley, pita bread, corn, baklava pastry
Supplementary:	Meat fats, olive and seed oils, honey, lemon juice, sour cream, turkish coffee and paste, apricot candies

JEWISH SELECTIONS

Diary products:	Milk, buttermilk, most all cheeses especially cottage cheese
Fruits and vegetables:	All vegetables, shav, latkes, borscht; all fruits with preference for dried fruits, oranges, apricots, apples
Meat, fish, eggs, legumes, nuts:	Kosher beef, lamb, veal, chicken, goose, turkey, duck, pigeon, carp, whitefish, caviar, smoked or salted fish, gefilte

	fish, lentils, dried beans, delicatessen corned beef, hot dogs, pastrami, salami, chopped liver
Bread, cereals, grains, pasta, rice:	Brown and white rice, rye, pumpernickel breads, rolls with seeds, challah, matzo, farfel, kasha, bagel, blintzes, bialys, matzo balls, strudel, cheesecake, macroons, sponge cake
Supplementary:	Butter, shmaltz (chicken fat), cream cheese, sour cream, vegetable oil, wine, kosher pickles, preserves

VEGETARIAN SELECTIONS

Diary products:	All milks, cheeses, ice cream, yogurt
Fruits and vegetables:	All fresh, canned, frozen, dried fruits and vegetables
Meat, fish, eggs, legumes, nuts:	No meat, fish or poultry; allowed are eggs, nuts, legumes (especially soybeans); some allow fish in their diet
Bread, cereals, grains, pasta, rice:	All breads with emphasis on whole wheat type, whole grain cereals
Supplementary:	Avoid fats, sweets; other supplements allowed

CHAPTER VII
PROCEDURES TO PROVIDE NUTRITION

ORAL FEEDINGS

Adequate nutritional intake by the elderly is influenced by physiological and psychosocial problems.

Problems with teeth and/or dentures

Sore oral cavity, dry mouth

Deteriorating oral structures

Chewing and swallowing problems, loss of tongue strength

Inability to use and manipulate eating utensils

Taste and smell deficits, visual problems

Nausea, vomiting, anorexia, dyspnea

Inflammatory conditions of the gastrointestinal tract

Tumors of the gastrointestinal tract

Effect of medications on nutrition

Psychosocial problems include:

Dementia (confusion, disorientation, forgetfulness)

Grieving, depression

Isolation, loneliness

Refusal to eat

Compliance with special dietary requirements

Insomnia

Ignorance of cultural dietary pattern

FEEDING / ASSISTING WITH MEAL

See "Age-Related Tips to Promote Nutrition"

Feeding can develop into a problem for both client and staff responsible for feeding or assisting to feed meals. Steps to follow that may lead to a successful experience are:

— Assist client to use bathroom, commode before meals

— Assist to wash hands before meals

— Position upright or sitting in chair preferably in a communal setting or, if alone, with a radio or TV on

— Be sure to offer correct diet with foods that are palatable and culturally appropriate

— Place tray in front of and within reach of client at appropriate height, check temperature of foods

— Show patience, smile, avoid rushing attitude

— For client needing assistance, cut meat in small bite sizes, open cartons and packages and pour, spread or sprinkle as appropriate

— Provide assistive utensils for self-feeding

— Praise all efforts and encourage to continue independent feeding

— If feeding, offer small bits of each food and allow to chew and swallow, offer fluids between bites if desired; give client the opportunity to select order of food offered and amounts

— If refused to be fed, allow to feed self no matter how awkward; protect clothing from spills

— Prevent any interruptions at mealtime

— Talk and socialize with client when feeding

— Always explain what foods are presented and cater to individual preferences and culturally symbolic foods when possible

USE OF ASSISTIVE AIDS

— Assess physical limitations and causes

— Assess use of dominant hand, arm or other hand and arm, hand-mouth coordination

— Provide assistive aids as appropriate: Suction dishes, cups that don't tip and spill

— Tongs to reach for food

— Lap board if in wheelchair

— Grip with large handle to fit carton for easy pouring

— Extension handles and adjustable shafts on forks, spoons and knives; swivel spoon or fork, rocker knife

— Built-up utensils with foam and tape

— Cuff-mounted utensils that slip over the hand eliminating the need to grasp utensils

— Glass holder; adhesive tape on glass to prevent slipping

— Tilting glass holder and straw to allow for holding straw while glass is stationary

— Sandwich holder, bumper guard dishes to assist food to be pushed onto a fork or spoon

— Non-slip placemats, napkin tucked at neckline

NASOGASTRIC / GASTROSTOMY FEEDINGS

Tube feedings are administered into the stomach through a tube inserted into the nose (nasogastric) or one that is surgically implanted through the abdominal wall (gastrostomy). The same feeding formulae are used for both feeding methods. These methods are used when a client is unable to ingest food orally but still maintains bowel function. Most likely elderly clients are those with dental and oral structure deterioration problems, gastrointestinal disease, paralysis, comatose, anorexia and depression or extreme weakness.

TYPES OF TUBES

— Keofeed tube: Silicone rubber tube, soft and pliable with a column of mercury at the distal end as a weight

— Dobbhoff tube: Polyurethane tube with a mercury weight that is passed into the duodenum or jejunum

— Med Pro tube: Silicone rubber tube of a smaller lumen that requires a pump to administer feedings

— Levin tube: Larger tube that is more irritating to the mucosa and causes swallowing difficulties

NASOGASTRIC TUBE INSERTION

— Assess client's nares for deviation and patency, gag reflex

— Assess nutritional status, long or short term feedings, continuous or intermittent feedings

— Assemble and prepare supplies; place soft tube in ice water and firm tube in warm water

— Position in sitting or high-Fowler's; place pillow behind shoulders

— Place towel over chest and have client hold basin or glass of water with straw

— Measure tube from tip of nose to earlobe to xyphoid process and mark with tape

— Dip prelubricated tube tip in water or lubricate with water soluble lubricant 3-4 inches from tip

— Coil tube around hand and gently and steadily insert tip of tube into nares in a downward and lateral movement

— Rotate tube during insertion and when pharynx is reached, instruct to swallow a small amount of water while continuing to insert the tube; insert with each swallow until marked length is reached

— Check pharynx, if gagging continues, with a flashlight and tongue blade as tubing may be coiled in back of mouth or trachea

— Check placement by aspirating gastric contents with a syringe or inject air through tube and listen to stomach with stethoscope for swooshing sounds

— Secure tube in place with the least amount of pressure to the nasal mucosa

— For long term nasogastric feedings, rotate nares to prevent damage to mucosa from prolonged pressure and irritation

— Provide thorough mouth care 3-4 times/day for dryness and discomfort

— Apply protective ointment to nares and lips to decrease irritation; change tape daily or if wet or loose

— Use throat sprays or lozenges to relieve throat discomfort; provide chewing gum or hard candy if permitted

— For gastrostomy care, use sterile technique for dressing changes or any wound cleansing procedures

— If gastrostomy tube is removed between feedings, wash in warm, soapy water, rinse, dry and store in clean bag until next feeding

— For gastrostomy tube insertion, remove dressing from stoma, dip tip of tube in water and gently insert into stoma 4-6 inches (remove and reinsert at a different angle if resistance is met), clamp or cap tubing until ready to administer feeding

TYPES OF FORMULA

— Institutional or blenderized formulated feeding: Prepared each day usually from a milk base and strained. Must be refrigerated; used in long term tube feeding. It usually contains evaporated milk, cooked farina, powdered egg, pureed liver or meat, orange juice, cooked vegetable in combination to total approximately 1050 kcal, 65 Gm protein, 77 Gm carbohydrate, 51 Gm fat and vitamins and minerals

— Commercially prepared formulated feeding: Also known

as formula diets for medical use, dietary supplements, enteral feedings, they are available in cans in liquid form or packages in powder form. They are available with the major nutrients of protein, carbohydrate or fat or for specific medical conditions such as renal failure, COPD, liver disfunction, low sodium, to supply additional calories, to supply meal replacements (complete defined formula), those that require a minimum of digestion (pre-digested)

COMMON COMMERCIAL FEEDINGS

Name	Uses	Preparation	Total Calories/L
Ensure	Oral or Tube	Canned/No preparation	1060/Lactose free
Osmolite	Oral or Tube	Canned/No preparation	1060 Lactose free Low osmolality
Sustacal	Oral or Tube	Canned and powdered	1000
Vital	Oral or Tube	Powdered 1 package: 8 1/2 oz water	1000/Lactose free Low residue
Citrotein	Oral or Tube	Powdered 1/4 cup: 1/4 cup water	533/Lactose free Low residue

High Protein: Gevral = 0.9 kcal/ml; EMF = 2.0 kcal/ml

High Carbohydrate: Hycal = 2.3 kcal/ml; Sumacal = 2.78 kcal/ml

High Fat: Lipomul-Oral = 6.0 kcal/ml; MCT Oil - 8.30 kcal/ml

Low Salt: Lonalac = 0.67 kcal/ml

Low Protein: Amin-Aid = 4.69 kcal/Gm

High Calorie, Low Sodium: Liprotein = 5.44 kcal/Gm

High Protein: Probana = 0.67 kcal/ml

FORMULA PREPARATION

Liquid:

— Check container for cracks, leaks and expiration date

— Rinse top of can or bottle and dry with paper toweling

— Open container and pour proper amount into feeding container or a graduated container if measurement is necessary

152

— Close feeding container; refrigerate amount not used

— If administering via a syringe barrel by gravity, take the measured amount in the graduated container to client

— If commercially prepared, give at room temperature; if institution prepared, remove from regrigerator 15 minutes before administration or immerse in warm water for short period of time (warmth encourages bacterial growth in formula so these procedures may be modified)

Powdered:

— Gradually add appropriate amount of powder to appropriate amount of liquid and mix to dissolve (may use clean blender)

— Prepare only the amount needed for 24 hours

— Pour proper amount into feeding container or graduated container if using syringe barrel to administer by gravity

— Close feeding container; cover and refrigerate mixture not used and label with date and time of preparation

— Follow same warming instructions as for liquid formula that has been refrigerated before subsequent feedings

— If medication given per tube, discontinue any continuous feedings 15 minutes before administration: crush tablet, empty capsule in some tap water or prepare measured liquid, check for tube placement and pour measured liquid, check for tube placement and pour medication into plunger while holding it 6 inches above nose and allow to rest for 15 minutes, reconnect continuous feedings or clamp tube

ADMINISTRATION OF FEEDINGS

Check for type of formula, feeding times, amount and frequency, method of administration (gravity or pump)

— Position in semi-Fowler's and place towel over chest

— Unclamp or uncap feeding tube and check placement in stomach

— Aspirate for residual and withold if more than 150 ml

— Return aspirate and connect barrel of asepto syringe to feeding tube

— Flush with 30 ml tap water and follow with addition of formula into syringe or funnel and raise 12-18 inches above stomach level and allow to flow; keep adding feeding to barrel or funnel before it empties until prescribed amount given

— Flush with 30-60 ml tap water before formula completed and reclamp or recap feeding tube

— Avoid any pressure to feeding and maintain position for 30 minutes following feeding

— If feedings continuous, pour prepared formula into container and close top; attach administration set to container and remove air before attaching to feeding tube; regulate drop rate with or without use of infusion pump; check for residual periodically and flush feeding tube with 30 ml tap water every 8-12 hours

— Place ice in ice container attached to formula container and replace as needed

COMPLICATIONS OF TUBE FEEDINGS

— Bacterial contamination as result of improper handling or storage

— Feeding at a rapid rate causing distention and bloating

— Delayed gastric emptying as motility decreased and too much formula is given causing nausea

— Improper placement of tube which may result in aspiration

— Feeding that is too cold causing increased emptying of stomach and diarrhea

— High osmolarity causing diarrhea and dehydration

— High lactose concentration causing diarrhea and dehydration if lactose intolerance present

— Allergic reaction

TOTAL PARENTERAL NUTRITION

Total parenteral nutrition (TPN) is the intravenous administration of nutrients that provides a complete support for long periods of time when oral, tube or intravenous therapy is inadequate or contraindicated. The process provides all of the caloric and nutritional requirements in a hypertonic solution via a large vien, usually the subclavian. Fat emulsion (intrapipids) is administered via subcuatenous vien. The catheter for TPN is surgically placed and anchored by the physician and maintained with strict sterile technique.

INDICATIONS FOR TPN

— Malnutrition, cachexia resulting from chronic diseases

— Preparation for surgery if nutritional status poor

— Inflammatory diseases of intestinal tract

— Inadequate or inability to ingest foods or absorb nutrients

Composition of Solutions

TPN solution (1 liter)-possible inclusions:

200 Gm	Glucose
42.5 Gm	Amino Acids
50 mEq	Sodium
10 mEq	Calcium
10 mM	Phosphate
35 mEq	Potassium
8 mEq	Magnesium
0.1 mg	Manganese
1.0 mg	Zinc
0.4 mg	Copper
4 mcg	Chromium
0.5 mg	Folic Acid
550 mg	Ascorbic Acid
	B Complex vitamins
3.5 ml	Multivitamin preparation added/week

Calories calculated to specific need of client

Intralipid solution:

2.5 Gm/kg/day is usual amount administered
Solution composed of soybean oil, egg yolk phosphatide and glycerol
Included in TPN regimen if client needs long term therapy (2 weeks
or more) and requirement cannot be met by feedings, however, used
with caution in those with pancreas, liver, pulmonary disorders

Complications

— Glucose metabolism: Hyperglycemia resulting from excessive rate of infusion, excessive total load of infusion,
inadequate or persistent insulin response

— Amino acid metabolism: Metabolic acidosis resulting
from excessive chloride and monohydrochloride content of
amino acid solutions; azotemia resulting from excessive
amino acid infusion

— Essential fatty acid deficiency: Thrombocytopenia, poor
wound healing resulting from inadequate fatty acids

— Calcium, phosphorus metabolism: Hypophosphatemia
and hypocalcemia resulting from inadequate administration in TPN solution

— Hypervitaminosis/hypovitaminosis: Excessive or deficient administration of vitamins

Care and Maintenance of TPN

— Vital signs every 4-8 hours, temperature every 4 hours

— Weight every day or every other day

— Monitor for urinary glucose every 4 hours

— Monitor glucose, potassium, sodium, calcium, protein,
lipid levels and nitrogen balance

— Change solution and tubing when appropriate

— Change dressing at insertion site when needed

— Monitor drop rate, change when necessary

— Monitor catheter and tubing patency

INTRAVENOUS FLUID THERAPY

Intravenous replacement and maintenance of fluid by peripheral infusion.

It is usually reserved for short term nutritional support for the administration of fluid, calories (glucose) and mineral salts (sodium chloride, potassium, magnesium, calcium and phosphate) according to specific client needs. One liter of 5% dextrose in water (D5W) equals 200 kcal and one liter of 10% dextrose in water (D10W) equals 400 kcal. An isotonic solution given is 5% dextrose in normal saline (D5NS).

Common IV Solutions

Solution	Contents	Uses
D5W (5% dextrose in water)	5Gm dextrose/100ml	Provides fluids; prevents dehydration
D5 1/2NS (5% dextrose in 0.45% normal saline)	5 Gm dextrose/100 ml	Replaces fluid and sodium losses; promotes diuresis
NS (0.9% sodium chloride)	14 mEq/L sodium 154 mEq/L chloride	Fluid losses
Ringers solution	14 mEq/L sodium 155 mEq/L chloride 4 mEq/L potassium 4 mEq/L calcium	Replaces fluid and electrolytes in vomiting or diarrhea dehydration
Lactated ringers	130 mEq/L sodium 109 mEq/L chloride 4 mEq/L potassium 3 mEq/L calcium	Dehydration Restoration of fluid balance

Indications

— Vomiting, diarrhea, excessive fluid losses from other routes

— Prevention of dehydration

— Need for electrolyte replacement

— Need to restore plasma volume

— Inability to take fluids orally

— Increased fluid requirements from fever, increased metabolism

Care and Maintenance

— Calculate I&O to determine fluid needs

— Calculate drip rate correctly and maintain prescribed rate

— Change solution and tubing when necessary

— Change IV sites when needed

— Monitor infusion site for infiltration (pain, swelling, leakage around insertion site, lack of flow)

— Monitor for fluid and elctrolyte imbalances

Calculation of Drip Rate

The rate is calculated using the amount of fluid to be infused, amount of time to infuse the fluid, number of drops/ml delivered by the infusion set (drop factor)

An order for 1 L D5W to run at 120 ml/hour is calculated as follows:

Drop factor of set is 15 drops/ml

Total amount $\quad x \quad$ Drop factor = Drops/minute

Minutes to infuse

$$\frac{120\ ml}{60\ minutes} \times 15\ \text{drops}/\text{ml} = \frac{1800}{15} = 120\ \text{drops}/\text{hour}$$

Sets may be calibrated in 10, 15 or 60 drops/ml

CHAPTER VIII
DRUGS RELATED TO NUTRITION AND DIET THERAPY AND INTERACTIONS

ANALGESICS
aspirin (Bayer)
acetaminophen (Tylenol)
codeine (Methylmorphine)- narcotic analgesic
oxycodone (Percodan)- narcotic analgesic

Action:	Binds with receptors of CNS to relieve pain
Indications:	Mild, moderate pain relief
Effect on Nutrition:	Aspirin (nausea, vomiting, gastro-intestinal distress, bleeding, reduces folate and vitamin C); narcotic analgesic (nausea, vomiting, constipation, dry mouth, biliary tract spasms)

ANTACIDS
aluminum hydroxide (Amphojel)
magaldrate (Riopan)
magnesium hydroxide (Milk of Magnesia)
sodium bicarbonate (Baking Soda)

Action:	Neutralizing action to reduce gastric acid concentration by raising pH of secretions
	In high doses, magnesium hydroxide acts as a laxative
Indications:	Gastritis, hiatal hernia with esophageal reflux, peptic ulcer; magnesium hydroxide for short term treatment of constipation
Effect on Nutrition:	Reduced phosphate and vitamin A absorption by aluminium hydroxide; reduced iron, phosphate absorption by magnesium preparations; steatorrhea by calcium carbonate; sodium content of bicarbonate causing edema; excessive milk intake when taking antacids causes hypercalcemia or milk-alkali syndrome; decreased thiamine activity in presence of systemic alkalosis in chronic use of antacids

ANTICHOLINERGICS
atropine sulfate (Atropine)
belladonna
propantheline bromide (Pro-Banthine)

Action:	Reduces smooth muscle contractions in stomach, intestinal tract, ureters, urinary bladder, gallbladder and bile ducts
Indications:	Peptic ulcer, pylorospasm, gastrointestinal hypermotility, irritable bowel, biliary spastic disorders
Effect on Nutrition:	Slows gastric emptying by decreasing peristaltic action; increases absorption of riboflavin; dry mouth, constipation and urinary retention, dysphagia, loss of taste, nausea, vomiting, bloated feeling

ANTICOAGULANTS
dicumarol (Bishydroxycoumarin)

warafin sodium (Coumadin)

Action:	Depresses hepatic synthesis of vitamin K dependent coagulation factors (II, VII, IX, X) to prevent blood clotting
Indications:	Deep venous thrombosis, myocardial infarction, emboli
Effect on Nutrition:	Vitamin K deficiency; anorexia, nausea vomiting, diarrhea, steatorrhea, stomatitis; excessive ingestion of vitamin K food intake decreases effect on anticoagulant

ANTICONVULSANTS/SEDATIVES
phenobarbital (Luminal)

phenytoin (Dilantin)

valproic acid (Depakene)

Action:	Reduced voltage, frequency and spread of electrical discharges in brain causing inhibition of seizure acthvity; sedation
Indications:	Prevent or treat seizures
Effect on Nutrition:	Folic acid and vitamin D deficiencies (decreased absorption); vitamin K deficiency by catabolism; reduced absorption of B_{12}, xylose; decreased blood levels of Ca, Mg; increased blood levels of Cu; gingival hyperplasia, nausea, vomiting, constipation, dysphagia, loss of taste, weight loss, megoblastic anemia

ANTIDEPRESSANTS
amitriptyline (Elavil)

imipramine (Tofranil)

Action:	Restoration of neurotransmitters to control depression (serotonin and norepinephrine)
Indications:	Endogenous depression treatment; reactive depression
Effect on Nutrition:	Stimulate appetite, weight gain, nausea, vomiting, dry mouth, epigastric distress, metallic taste all of which may cause weight loss

ANTIDIARRHEALS
diphenoxylate with atropine (Lomotil)

kaolin and pectin (Kaopectate)

Action:	Reduces gastrointestinal motility by inhibiting mucosal receptors; kaolin and pectin acts as an absorbent and demulcent to consolidate feces
Indications:	Diarrhea management
Effect on Nutrition:	Nausea, vomiting, anorexia, dry mouth, abdominal distention, paralytic ileus; loss of fluid and nutrients before absorption; fluid and electrolyte imbalance

ANTIEMETICS
dimenhydrinate (Dramamine)

promethazine (Phenergan)

prochlorperazine (Compazine)

Action:	Depresses chemoreceptor zone in medulla
Indications:	Nausea and vomiting management
Effect on Nutrition:	Anorexia, constipation or diarrhea, dry mouth; inability to ingest foods, fluids resulting in nutritional deficiencies and fluid and electrolyte imbalances

ANTIFLATULANTS
simethicone (Gas-X)

Action:	Defoams gastric juice by coalescing gas bubbles
Indications:	Flatulence and gastric bloating
Effect on Nutrition:	None; relieves gas discomfort

ANTIHYPERTENSIVES
methyldopa (Aldomet)

hydralazine (Apresoline)

captopril (Capoten)

reserpine (Serpasil)

Action:	Acts on smooth muscle resulting in vasodilation of arteries and reduced peripheral resistance; inhibits angiotensin- converting enzyme resulting in lowered peripheral resistance
Indications:	Hypertension
Effect on Nutrition:	Anorexia, nausea, vomiting, diarrhea, dry mouth, increased gastric motility; increased excretion of Mg and vitamin B_6 (pyridoxine); requires increases in B_{12} and folate

ANTI-INFLAMMATORY AGENTS

colchicine (Novocolchine)

prednisone (Deltasone)

aspirin (Bayer)

ibuprofen (Motrin)

indomethacin (Indocin)

Action:	Inhibits prostoglandin biosynthesis (aspirin, ibuprofen, indomethacin); crosses cell membrane and complexes to increase body defenses (prednisone), treatment of inflammatory disorders, arthritis and others (ibuprofen, et al)
Effect on Nutrition:	colchicine (decreased absorption of B_{12}, fats, nitrogen, sodium, potassium, calcium, cholesterol, iron, lactose, sucrose, carotene; absorptive and intestinal wall damage); prednisone and other corticosteroids (increased appetite, weight gain, decreased absorption of calcium, iron, phosphorus, glucose tolerance, muscle protein, renal sodium loss; increased fat and cholesterol absorption, vitamin D metabolism, calcium, magnesium, zinc, potassium, vitamin C excretion; increased need for vitamin B_6 caused by increased conversion of tryptophan; poor wound healing, negative nitrogen balance, edema, gastric inflammation and ulcer, osteoporosis); ibuprofen and other nonsteroidals (gastrointestinal bleeding, increased thiamin and vitamin C excretion, decreased iron absorption and vitamin C metabolism)

ANTILIPEMICS
cholestryamine (Questran)
clofibrate (Novofibrate)
probucol (Loreice)

Action:	Reduces low density lipoprotein (LDL) by inhibiting cholesterol synthesis
Indications:	Hyperlipoproteinemia, type II or III
Effect on Nutrition:	cholestyramine (malabsorption of cholesterol, vitamins A, D, K, B_{12}, folate, iron, calcium, monosaccharides, increases calcium excretion); clofibrate (decreased absorption of A, D, K, B_{12}, sugar, carotene, iron electrolyes, triglycerides; increased excretion of sterols; altered taste, anorexia, inhibited carbohydrate digestion, abnormal muscle metabolism)

ANTIMICROBIALS
cephalosporins, penicillins, erythromycins, tetracyclines, aminoglycosides, sulfonamides

Action:	Binds to proteins on cell wall to inhibit wall synthesis of microorganisms; sulfonamides act by interfering with folic acid synthesis needed for growth of microorganisms
Effect on Nutrition:	Loss of appetite, diarrhea with loss of intestinal flora, decreased intestinal synthesis of B vitamins and vitamin K, protein synthesis, anemia with altered hemoglobin synthesis, steatorrhea with intestinal mucosa damage and decreased enzymes to act on fat, cholesterol and bile acids, decreased pancreatic enzymes and absorption of triglycerides, disaccharides, nitrogen, vitamins A, K, B_{12}, iron, calciuml, potassium; after taste, sodium content, may chelate with minerals or decrease absorption of minerals if taken with milk, antacids or iron; the many drugs in these categories may result in one or more of the above effects. Overall, when antimicrobials are administered, vitamins and minerals may have to be supplemented

166

ANTINEOPLASTICS
Antibiotics, hormones, antimetabolites, alkylating agents, corticosteroids, vinca alkaloids, cytotoxic agents

Action:	Prevents cell wall synthesis (antibiotics); blocks action of enzymes essential to RNA and DNA synthesis causing death of cells (antimetabolites); inhibits RNA, DNA and protein synthesis (alkylating agents); arrests mitosis and inhibits cell division (vinca alkaloids); palliative therapy (hormones); anti-inflammatory agent (corticosteroids)
Indications:	Chemotherapy for malignant neoplasm
Effect on Nutrition:	Nausea, vomiting, anorexia, stomatitis, buccal ulceration, glossitis, gum inflammation causing decreased intake; altered taste, gastrointestinal tract inflammation causing decreased absorption of nutrients, bleeding, diarrhea; abnormal liver function, anemia; malabsorption of folate, fat xylose, B_{12}; negative protein balance

DIGESTANTS
pancreatin (Dizymes)

Action:	Assists in digestion of protein, carbohydrate and fat
Indications:	Digestive aid in pancreatitis or pancreas deficiency
Effect on Nutrition:	Inhibits absorption of iron, anorexia, nausea, vomiting

DIURETICS
furosemide (Lasix)
hydrochlorothiazide (Hydro-Diuril)
ethacrynic acid (Edecrin)

Action:	Enhances secretion of body fluids
Indications:	Edema associated with renal, cardiac, liver disease
Effect on Nutrition:	Promotes excretion of Na, Cl, K, Mg resulting in electrolyte imbalance; fluid imbalance and dehydration; increases excretion of vitamin B (thiamin), vitamin B_2 (riboflavin), zinc, folate

HEMATINICS
ferrous sulfate (Feosol)

Action:	Supplements or replaces iron to correct erythropoietic problems
Indications:	Iron-deficiency anemia treatment
Effect on Nutrition:	Lack of iron and need for dietary replacement, nausea, vomiting; absorption increased by vitamin C (ascorbic acid)

HISTAMINE BLOCKERS
cimetidine (Tagamet)

ranitidine (Zantac)

Action:	Suppresses gastric acid and pepsin secretion
Indications:	Gastritis, peptic ulcer
Effect on Nutrition:	May cause constipation or diarrhea; changes in digestion with decreased HCl

HORMONES
insulin

Action:	Lowers blood glucose levels
Indication:	Diabetes mellitus
Effect on Nutrition:	Increases appetite, weight gain

HYPOGLYCEMICS
glipizide (Glucetrol)

glyburide (Micronase)

Action:	Stimulate function of beta cells in pancreas to secrete insulin and reduces glucagon levels
Indications:	Diabetes mellitus Type II (NIDDM)
Effect on Nutrition:	Adjunct to dietary intake to control hyperglycemia by aiding digestion of carbohydrates

LAXATIVES/CATHARTICS/STOOL SOFTENERS/ BULK LAXATIVES
mineral oil

phenolphthalein (Correctol, Ex-Lax)

magnesium sulfate (Milk of Magnesia)

ducosate (Surfax, Colace)

psyllium (Metamucil)

Action:	Relieves constipation by providing bulk to feces; lowering surface tension to allow water and fats to mix with and soften feces; increases peristalis by irritation to mucosa

Indications: Short term constipation treatment

Effect on Nutrition: Increased motility and decreased absorption of glucose by intestine, steatorrhea, losses of Na, K, albumin with excessive use; malabsorption of fat soluble vitamins with use of mineral oil; decreased Ca and vitamin D absorption and protein loss with use of phenolphthalein

REPLACEMENT AGENTS
potassium chloride (K-Lyte)
calcium gluconate (Kalcinate)
multivitamin (Vicon-Forte)

Action: Replaces lost electrolytes;

Indications: Menopausal women, diuretic therapy, malnutrition

Effects on Nutrition: Decreases absorption of vitamin B_{12}

TRANQUILIZERS
chlordiazepoxide (Librium)
diazepam (Valium)
lorazepam (Ativan)

Action: Inhibits neurotransmitter action of CNS

Indications: Management of anxiety disorders for short term use

Effect on Nutrition: Weight gain as appetite increases, hyperglycemia, glucosuria, hypercholesterolemia

MISCELLANEOUS
alcohol
levodopa (L-Dopa)-Antiparkinsonian
digitalis (Digoxin)-Cardiac glycoside

Action: Digitalis slows and strengthens cardiac contractions; levodopa restores dopamine in extrapyramidal centers; alcohol depresses CNS

Indications: Parkinson's disease, heart failure

Effect on Nutrition: Digitalis decreases glucose absorption and increases Ca and Mg excretion; levodopa decreases Na and K levels, may need higher levels of folate and vitamin B_{12}, B_6 and lower intake of proteins; alcohol leads to malnutrition and decreased absorption of glucose, fat, vitamins B_{12}, B_1; folate and increased excretion of Mg, Ca and zinc

CHAPTER IX
Diagnostic Procedures and Laboratory Tests Related to the Gastrointestinal System and Nutrition

DIAGNOSTIC PROCEDURES

Cystoscopy (Cystograph)
Visualization of the bladder wall and urethra by insertion of a lighted telescopic lens attached to a tubular scope. Instillation of a contrast dye into the bladder through a catheter and x-rays taken may follow cystoscopy. Reveals calculi or tumor of the urinary bladder

Esophageal Studies (Manometry)
Measurement of esophageal acidity, esophageal sphincter pressure, differentiate between esophagitis and cardiac conditions.
Reveals gastroesophageal reflux, duration and strength of esophageal peristalsis in achalasia and esophagitis.

Flat Plate (Radiography)
Radiology examination of the abdominal organs by x-ray
Reveals abdominal masses, bowel obstruction or ascites

Gallbladder Series (Cholecystography)
Radiology examination to view the gallbladder after ingestion of radiopaque tablets (iopanic acid) with water the evening before the test. A fat meal may be given after the fasting x-rays are taken and additional films taken at intervals to determine how fast the gallbladder expels the dye. Reveals gallbladder and presence of cholelithiasis, cholecystitis, cystic duct obstruction, neoplasm of the gallbladder

Lower Gastrointestinal Series (Barium Enema)
Radiology examination including fluoroscopy to view the colon after administration of a contrast medium enema. Air studies may also be done after inserting air into the colon following the elimination of the contrast medium. Reveals colon and presence of diverticular disease, colitis, polyps, neoplasms

Nuclear Imaging (Radionuclide Scan)
Imaging of the liver, pancreas and gallbladder, using an x-ray beam produced by a computerized scanner of different body sections at different angles after a radioactive isotope is injected intravenously. Reveals tumors, cysts, or enlargement of the organs and other abnormalities

Proctosigmoidoscopy (Proctoscopy)

Visual examination to view the rectum and sigmoid colon after insertion of a rigid or flexible lighted endoscope. Reveals the mucosa and structure of the rectum and lower sigmoid and presence of polyps, internal hemorrhoids, fissure, fistula, inflammation, abscess, neoplasms

Ultrasound (Echography, Sonography)

Visualization of the abdomen, liver, gallbladder and intestines using high-frequency sound waves that pass through the body and are recorded on a screen (oscilloscope) as they are echoed or bounced back. Abnormalities are confirmed by nuclear imaging or computerized tomography. Reveals masses of the abdomen, tumors or cirrhosis of the liver, gallstones of the gallbladder and biliary obstruction, tumor of the pancreas.

Upper Gastrointestinal Series (Barium Swallow)

Radiology examination including fluoroscopy to view the stomach after ingestion of a contrast medium (barium sulfate). Small bowel radiology examination to view the small intestine every 20 minutes after a contrast medium is taken until the medium reaches the end of the ileum.

Reveals esophagus, stomach and small intestines and presence of hiatal hernia, peptic ulcer, diverticula of stomach or duodenum, esophageal varices, gastritis, gastroenteritis, neoplasms

LABORATORY TESTS

BLOOD TESTS

Alanine Aminotransferase (ALT, SGPT)
5-35 U/ml (Frankel)
An enzyme in the liver revealing liver destruction (hepatitis, cirrhosis, cancer) when levels are increased

Aldosterone
1-9 ng/dl (RIA)
A mineralocorticoid produced by the adrenal cortex to regulate water, Na and K balance. Increases caused by dehydration, Na deficit and decreases by fluid overload, Na excess

Alkaline Phosphatase (ALP)
2-4 U/dl (Bodansky)
An enzyme in the liver and bone revealing liver damage, biliary disease (cancer, cirrhosis, hepatitis, jaundice) when levels are increased

Ammonia
80-110 mcg/dl (Method dependent)
A by-product of protein metabolism resulting from bacterial action in the intestine with most circulated to the liver and converted to urea which is excreted by the kidneys. Reveals liver failure if level increased and renal failure if decreased

Amylase
60-160 Somogyi U/dl
An enzyme of the pancreas, liver and salivary gland involved in digestion of starches to sugar. Reveals pancreas diseases, both chronic and acute

Bilirubin (Total and Direct)
Total: 0.1-1.2 mg/dl
Direct: 0.1-0.3 mg/dl
A product of hemoglobin breakdown that is transported to the liver and changed to bilirubin which is excreted in the bile. Increases in direct bilirubin is caused by obstructive jaundice from stones or tumor in the hepatobiliary system

Blood Urea Nitrogen (BUN)
Female: 8-20 mg/dl
Male: 10-25 mg/dl
A product (urea) of protein metabolism excreted by the kidneys. Reveals malnutrition, overhydration and liver damage with increased levels and renal failure or deficiency, dehydration with decreases

Calcium (Ca)
4.5-5.5 mEq/L or 9-11 mg/dl
A mineral found in the bones and teeth with 50% ionized (Ca) as an electrolyte. Levels decreased in diarrhea, malabsorption disorders, laxative abuse, reduced vitamin D intake and may result in tetany

Chloride (Cl)
95-105 mEq/L
An anion (Cl) found in the extracellular fluid that is involved in maintaining water balance and osmolality of body fluids. Levels decreased in vomiting, diarrhea, gastroenteritis and colitis and with reduced Na and K and increased in dehydration, kidney dysfunction and increased Na

Cholesterol
150-200 mg/dl
A lipid synthesized by the liver. Levels used to determine liver function, atherosclerosis and coronary artery disease. Increases due to high dietary intake or a genetic factor

Copper (Cu)
Female: 80-155 mcg/dl
Male: 70-140 mcg/dl
An element needed for synthesis of hemoglobin. Protein malnutrition causes decreased levels and anemia and cancer of the liver, stomach, colon increases levels

D-xylose Absorption Test
30-58 mg/dl/2 hours; Urine Value of 16-33% of amount of D-xylose ingested
A test to determine small intestine absorption reveals celiac disease, enteritis

Gamma-Glutamyl Transferase (GGT)
Female: 5-25 IU/L
Male: 10-38 IU/L

An enzyme found in the liver and kidneys. Levels increased with liver dysfunction (cirrhosis, necrosis, hepatitis, cancer), alcoholism

Gastrin
40-200 pg/ml

A hormone secreted by the pyloric mucosa which stimulates HC1 secretion. Increased levels in pernicious anemia, gastritis, peptic ulcer, stomach cancer, cirrhosis of liver

Glucose (FBS)
60-100 mg/dl in whole body; Postprandial of less than 120 mg/dl/2 hours.

The end product of digestion of carbohydrates and stored as glycogen in the liver and muscle tissue. Decreased levels are caused by too much insulin or inadequate intake and increased levels from an inadequate amount of or reduced effectiveness of insulin. Diabetes is indicated by an increase of 120 mg/dl or more and is further confirmed by a postprandial or glucose tolerance test

Glucose Tolerance Test (GTT)
Fasting: 60-100 mg/dl in whole blood

30 minutes: Less than 150 mg/dl

1 hour: Less than 160 mg/dl

2 hours: Less than 115 mg/dl

Done as follow up test to blood glucose to determine presence of diabetes mellitus

Hematocrit (Hct)
Female: 37-48% or 37-48/dl

Male: 45-52% or 45-52/dl

Hct is the volume of packet RBC found in 1 dl blood. Low levels are found in anemias, vitamin deficiencies and increases levels in dehydration

Hemoblobin (Hgb)
Female: 12-16 Gm/dl

Male: 13-18 Gm/dl

Older adult: 10-17 Gm/dl

Hgb is a protein found in RBCs and composed of iron, the oxygen carrier component of the cell. Low levels are found in anemia and increased levels in dehydration

Iron (Fe)
50-150 mcg/dl

A mineral needed for hemoglobin synthesis in the bone marrow. Decreased levels are found in iron deficient anemia

Ketones
2-4 mg/dl

Products of fat metabolism. Levels increased in starvation, vomiting or diarrhea and diabetic ketoacidosis as fats are catabolized instead of carbohydrate metabolism

Lipase
2 U/ml or less

An enzyme secreted by the pancreas that is involved in fat digestion. Increases reveal pancrease disease (cancer, pancreatitis) and decreases found in hepatitis and late pancreatic cancer

Lipoproteins (Lipids)
Total: 400-800 mg/dl

Cholesterol: 150-200 mg/dl

Triglycerides: 10-190 mg/dl

Phospholipids: 150-380 mg/dl

These are lipids that are bound to protein. They may be separated by electrophoresis to reveal high-density lipoprotein (HDL), low-density lipoprotein (LDL) and very low-density lipoprotein (VLDL). The HDL, are considered good lipids while the LDL and VLDL contribute to coronary heart disease and general arthersclerosis

Magnesium (Mg)
1.5-2.0 mEq/L or 1.8-3.0 mg/dl

Found in the intracellular fluid and is necessary for neuromuscular activity. Some is converted to the cation Mg as an electrolyte and associated with activity of Ca and K. Decreased levels are associated with malnutrition (protein), malabsorption, alcoholism, cirrhosis of liver and increased levels with dehydration

Minerals/Elements
Chromium: 1-6 mcg/dl

Cobalt: 4.3 mcg/dl

Iodine: 4.8 mcg/dl

Maganese: 4-20 mcg/dl

Sulfur: 0.7-1.5 mEq/L

Zinc: 120 mcg/dl

See individual explanation of minerals and trace elements in Chapter 14 for function and body requirements. The more common minerals and electrolytes are covered specifically in this chapter.

Occult Blood (Feces)
Negative
Microscopic or frank blood in stools caused by gastrointestinal bleeding. Associated with peptic ulcer, colitis, esophageal varices, gastrointestinal cancer, diverticulitis

Phosphorus (P)
1.7-2.6 mEq/L or 2.5-4.5 mg/dl
An anion found in the intracellular fluid and exists mainly in an ionized form of phosphate (PO_4). Functions to metabolize carbohydrates and fats utilize B vitamins and maintain acid-base balance. Decreased levels in malnutrition, malabsorption disorders, alcoholism, vitamin D deficiency and with increases in Mg and Ca. Increases occur in renal failure, decreased Ca and increased vitamin D.

Potassium (K)
3.5-5.0 mEq/L
A mineral found mainly in the intracellular fluids in the form of an electrolyte (K). Levels are decreased in vomiting, diarrhea, dehydration, malnutrition and diuretic therapy and increased in renal failure and acidosis

Protein (Albumin, Globulin, Total)
Total: 6.0-8.0 Gm/dl
Albumin: 52-68% of total
Globulin: 23-48% of total
Albumin makes up the largest portion of the total protein and maintains the colloid osmotic pressure. The globulins also function to maintain osmotic pressure with the gamma globulins (antibodies) assisting in immunity processes. Levels are decreased in malnutrition, low protein diet, malabsorption, liver disease and increased in dehydration, vomiting, diarrhea

Red Blood Cell Count (RBC)
Female: 4-5.3 million/cu mm
Male: 4.4-6.0 million/cu mm
Older adult: 3-5 million/cu mm
The cell that contains hemoglobin and carries oxygen to the cells. Decreased values are associated with the anemias and the indices, mean corpuscular volmue (MCV), mean corpuscular hemoglobin (MCH),

and mean corpuscular hemoglobin concentration (MCHC) are used to identify the type of anemia

Schilling Test
A test for pernicious anemia by determining a deficiency in vitamin B_{12} caused by a defect in absorption or a deficiency of the intrinsic factor.

Sodium (Na)
135-145 mEq/L
A cation (Na) found mainly in the extracellular fluid and functions to maintain osmolality, acid-base balance, neuromuscular activity, enzyme activity. Decreased levels occur with vomiting, diarrhea, excessive perspiration and increased with dehydration, renal disease

Vitamins

Fat Soluble:
Vitamin A: 100-300 IU/100 Gm
Vitamin D: 65-165 IU/100 ml
Vitamin E: 1.11 mg/100 ml
Vitamin K: None available

Water Soluble:
Vitamin B_1 (thiamin): 1.3 mcg/dl
Vitamin B_2 (riboflavin): 6.6 mcg/dl
Vitamin B_3 (niacin): 0.42-0.84 mg/dl
Vitamin B_6 (pyridoxine): 11.2 mcg/dl
Vitamin B_{12} (cyanocobalamin): 0.08 mcg/dl
Vitamin C (ascorbic acid): 0.5-1.0 mg/dl
Folacin: 3.53 mcg/dl
Biotin: 1.23 mg/dl
Pantothenic Acid: 19-32 mcg/dl
See individual explanation of vitamins in Chapter IV for functions and body requirements

URINE TESTS

Urinalysis
pH: 4.6-8.0; Sp.gr.: 1.010-1.025; Protein: 0-15 mg/dl; Ketones: neg; Bilirubin: neg; Microscopic: neg or rare RBC, WBC, bacteria, casts, crystals, epithelial cells

Done to detect renal disease, metabolic disease; culture done to detect urinary tract infection with colonizations of 100,000/ml or more indication of presence of infection

Urobilinogen
0.3-3.5 mg/dl (Random Specimen)

A product of bilirubin conversion by intestinal bacteria that is excreted by the kidneys after it returns to the liver for manufacture into bile. Increased levels are found in liver disorders (hepatitis, cirrhosis) and decreased levels in cholelithiasis with biliary obstruction

Vitamins
Vitamin B_3 (nicotinamide): 0.6 or more mg/Gm creatinine

Vitamin B_6 (pyridoxine): 20 or more mcg/Gm creatinine

Vitamin B_2 (riboflavin): 80 or more mcg/Gm creatinine

Vitamin B_1 (thiamin): 65 or more mcg/Gm creatinine

Pantothenic acid: 200 or more mcg/dl

APPENDIX

GLOSSARY

Absorption: The process in which nutrients pass through the intestinal mucosa

Acid: A substance that releases hydrogen ions (H^+)

Acidosis: An increase of acid in the blood with a decrease in alkali

Alkalosis: A deficit of acid or an accumulation of alkali in the blood

Amino Acids: The units of which proteins are made

Anabolism: The process that metabolizes nutrients into complex substances for cell building and maintenance

Anion: An electrolyte with a negative charge

Anorexia: Loss of appetite

Base: A substance that accepts the hydrogen ion

Bolus: A food mass produced in the mouth and passed through the esophagus

Cachexia: An emaciated state of nutritional deficit associated with chronic illness

Calorie: The amount of heat or energy that raises the temperature of a gram of water 1 degree C

Carbohydrate: A substance composed of hydrogen, carbon and oxygen called a starch

Caries: The process of tooth decay

Catabolism: The process that metabolizes nutrients into smaller substances that is destructive to cell structure

Cation: An electrolyte with a positive charge

Cellulose: A part of plants that is not digestible by humans

Chyme: The liquified food during the process of digestion

Complete Protein: A protein that contains all of the essential proteins necessary for grwoth and maintenance of cells

Dehydration: An excess of fluid loss

Digestion: The process of the breakdown of foods to a form that can be absorbed by the gastrointestinal tract

Disaccharides: The linkage of two monosaccharides

Dysphagia: Difficult swallowing

Electrolyte: A substance that dissociates into ions when dissolved in water

Emesis: Vomiting

Enteral Feeding: Introducing nutrients into the gastrointestinal tract via a tube

Enzyme: A substance that acts as a catalyst for chemical reactions in the body

Essential Amino Acids: An amino acid that is not synthesized by the body and must be secured through dietary intake

Essential Fatty Acids: The polyunsaturated fats that are not synthesized by the body and must be secuared through dietary intake

Excretion: The process of waste elimination from the body

Fat: A substance composed of carbon, oxygen and hydrogen in water

Fatty Acids: The components of fats classified according to number of carbons and bonds between them

Fiber: The carbohydrate portion in plants and meats that cannot be digested by humans; also called bulk in the diet

Geriatric: The speciality in medicine concerned with diseases in the aged population

Gerontology: The study of aging

Globulin: A protein found in the blood plasma important in fighting infection

Glucose: A monosaccharide found in the blood available for immediate use and energy; also called dextrose

Glyceride: The simplest form of lipid consisting of glycerol and one or more fatty acids

Hormone: A substance produced by an endocrine gland that regulates body functions

Hypertonic: A fluid with higher osmolarity than body fluid

Hypotonic: A fluid with lower osmolarity than body fluid

Hypogeusia: Loss of taste sensation

Hyposmia: Loss of smell sensation

Ingestion: The process of eating or drinking

Ion: An atom with a positive or negative charge

Isotonic: A fluid with the same osmolarity as body fluid

Lipids: Fat and fat related substances

Malnutrition: An over or under nutritional state

Mastication: Chewing or grinding food

Metabolism: The total of all chemical processes in the body, anabolism and catabolism

Milk-Alkali Syndrome: Excessive intake of milk and an alkali resulting in alkalosis and renal dysfunction

Milliequivalents: A unit of measurement derived from the atomic weight of a substance divided by the valence of a substance

Minerals: Part of the body composition and the inorganic parts of food that are necessary for body function

Monosaccharides: A simple sugar that cannot be broken down by hydrolysis

Nitrogen balance: Equality of nitrogen intake and excretion

Nonessential Amino Acids: An amino acid that can be synthesized by the body

Nutrient: A substance in food that can be ingested, digested, absorbed and utrilized by the body

Osmosis: Movement of a solvent through a membrane from a less concentrated to a more concentrated solution

Peristalsis: The contraction and relaxation of the muscles of the gastrointestinal tract that moves a food bolus

Polysaccharide: A combination of monosaccharide units (10 or more)

Proteins: A nitrogen containing organic compound composed of amino acids

RDA: Recommended Daily Allowance

Regurgitation: Reflux of swallowed food into the mouth

Senescence: The process of aging or being elderly

Synthesis: The combination of substances to build or form a new substance

Triglyceride: A combination of three fatty acids and glycerol, also called a fat

Vitamins: Substances found in foods that are necessary to perform specific functions in metabolism

REFERENCES

Burnside, Irene M. *Nursing and the Aged.* 3rd ed., McGraw-Hill, New York, 1988.

Jaffe, M.S. and Melson, K.A. *Laboratory and Diagnostic Cards: Clinical Implications and Teaching.* C.V. Mosby Company, St. Louis, 1988.

Lewis, Clara M. *Nutrition and Nutritional Therapy in Nursing.* Appleton & Lange, Norwalk, 1986.

Lewis, S.M. and Collier, I.C. *Medical-Surgical Nursing: Assessment and Management of Clinical Problems.* 2nd ed., McGraw-Hill, New York, 1987.

Luke, Barbara. *Principles of Nutrition and Diet Therapy.* Little, Brown and Company, Boston, 1984.

North American Nursing Diagnosis Association. *Taxonomy I Revised With Official Nursing Diagnoses.* 1990.

Skidmore-Roth, Linda. *Mosby's Nursing Drug Reference.* Mosby/Yearbook, Inc., St. Louis, 1991.

Order Form

☐ Handbook of Long Term Care $15.95

☐ Nurse Assistant Handbook $15.95

☐ The Nurse's Survival Guide $19.95

☐ The Body in Brief $24.95

☐ The Nurse's Trivia Calendar $9.95

☐ Diagnostic and Laboratory Cards $21.95

☐ Procedure Cards for Clinical Use $19.95

☐ Geriatric Nutrition and Diet Therapy $17.95

☐ Pediatric Nursing Care Plans $27.95

☐ RN NCLEX Review Cards $23.95

☐ PN/VN Review Cards $23.95

☐ Geriatric Nursing Care Plans $27.95

Name _____

Address _____

City_____State_____Zip_____

Phone: (   )_____

☐ Visa ☐ Mastercard ☐ American Express
☐ Check/Money Order Attached

Card No. _____

Expiration Date _____

Signature:_____

Prices Subject to Change.
Please add $4.00 each for postage and handling.
Include your local sales tax.

Skidmore-Roth Publishing
1001 Wall Street
El Paso, Texas 79915
800-825-3150